Praise for the Second Edition of
Saving the Whole Woman

This updated version of Saving the Whole Woman is a breath of fresh air for thousands of women who have been diagnosed with uterine, bladder, or rectal prolapse. In truth, every woman should know the information in this book to help preserve her innate pelvic power.

CHRISTIANE NORTHRUP, MD
Author of Mother-Daughter Wisdom, The Wisdom of Menopause, and Women's Bodies, Women's Wisdom.

As a former gynecologic surgeon who came to see the error his ways, I passionately read 'Saving the Whole Woman'. Christine's work is medically accurate and will bring hope to millions of women suffering from pelvic organ prolapse and who want to avoid surgery. I hope mothers will share this work with their daughters to help them avoid the kind of childbirth experience that sets them up for problems later in life.

MICHEL ODENT, MD
Author of Primal Health and The Caesarean Director, Primal Health Research Center, London

Saving the Whole Woman is a one of a kind book. It provides natural, helpful solutions for women and takes away the stigma often associated with pelvic floor problems. The original research in this book could be lifesaving.

PEGGY O'MARA
Editor and Publisher Mothering Magazine

Saving the Whole Woman is a scathing account of the way the medical field uses and abuses women's bodies with regard to surgeries and procedures on the pelvic floor. These medical procedures parallel the mistreatment of women's bodies in the childbearing year, and in both cases money is often the motivating factor. Christine gives us hope by teaching us about our bodies and how we can prevent or solve problems without medical intervention. Give a copy to every woman you know, old or young.

JAN TRITTEN
Founder, Publisher & Editor-in-Chief of Midwifery Today magazine and The Birthkit newsletter

As a surgeon who became enlightened to natural health, I recommend avoiding surgery for the treatment of chronic disorders if there are natural approaches that work just as well, if not better. Christine Kent has made a major contribution to women by compiling a comprehensive research-supported natural approach to the common problems of pelvic organ prolapse and urinary incontinence. Any woman ready to take charge of her health needs to read this book!

CHRISTINE HORNER, MD FACS
Author of Waking the Warrior Goddess: Dr. Christine Horner's Program to Protect Against and Fight Breast Cancer, winner of the 2006 IPPY Award for "Best book in health, medicine, and nutrition".

Empowering women with accurate knowledge allows them to make informed decisions regarding their healthcare. For those women who are contemplating urogynecological surgery and for those healthcare practitioners who are advising these women, this new edition of Christine Kent's Saving the Whole Woman is an essential read. The evidence is substantial; restoring optimal posture and muscle function can prevent and reduce most pelvic organ prolapse and urinary incontinence. Surgery should not be your first treatment choice.

DIANE LEE
Physiotherapist & Author
The Pelvic Girdle

Christine Ann Kent is on a mission to expose the continuing tragedy of surgical mismanagement of pelvic problems. Her exhaustive and scholarly chronicle of the attempts to improve on female anatomy sends a serious warning: Avoid unnecessary or questionable surgery! Her detailed holistic approach to maintaining and restoring pelvic health reframes perceptions of female anatomy from "faulty" to "wondrous," and gives women the key to their own pelvic well-being.

PENNY SIMKIN, PT
Childbirth educator, doula and author including The Birth Partner and The Labor Progress Handbook

After over 36 years as an occupational therapist, I had an acute prolapse including difficulty with elimination. I greatly benefitted from Christine's exercises in only one session at The Whole Woman™ Center. Her book is very thorough anatomically, practical and honest about a very real problem to untold women. The sensible self-help instruction and lifestyle ideas are extremely helpful.

JAN HARRISON OTR/L
Monte Vista, CO

More Praise For
Saving the Whole Woman
First Edition

Saving the Whole Woman delves into the mysteries of the female body and the pelvic floor - and gives women the information they need to reclaim, honor, and protect the areas of our bodies that have too often been disowned and sacrified.

> CHRISTIANE NORTHRUP, M.D.
> *Author, Women's Bodies, Women's Wisdom (Bantam, 1998)and The Wisdom of Menopause (Bantam, 2001)*

The decision to undergo surgery of any kind is often difficult, so it is often useful to explore other alternatives before moving forward. In Saving the Whole Woman, Christine Kent provides a perspective of other options available to women who have been recommended to undergo pelvic surgery. This book may anger some and empower others.

> DEAN ORNISH, M.D.
> *Founder and President, Preventive Medicine Research Institute*
> *Clinical Professor of Medicine, University of California, San Francisco*
> *Author, Dr. Dean Ornish's Program for Reversing Heart Disease*

Christine Kent has written a definitive book on the holistic approach to pelvic organ prolapse and urinary incontinence for women. She exposes the risks and failures of surgical therapies and gives women alternatives in managing these issues and regaining a sense of their whole beings. Thank you Christine!

> LEE LIPSENTHAL, M.D.
> *President, The American Board of Holistic Medicine*

Every woman deserves and needs to know the vital information Christine has amassed in this book.

> ELIZABETH PLOURDE
> *Author, Your Guide to Hysterectomy, Ovary Removal & Hormone Replacement*

"I believe in the importance and the bravery of this book and hope that it will save women's lives and sanity."

> PHYLLIS CHESLER, PH.D.
> *Author, Women and Madness and Woman's Inhumanity to Woman*

"Women, especially around the time of menopause, are too often advised to have major gynecological surgery for minor conditions that can be significantly improved with natural alternatives. In Saving the Whole Woman, Christine Kent has made an important contribution to women's health literature by recounting her own story of unnecessary surgery and its effect upon her life. Her research of the medical information on pelvic organ prolapse and urinary incontinence is accurately and clearly presented and can serve as a warning to other women. Her critique of the lack of oversight or scientifically-based criteria for such surgery should be read by every woman and provider of women's health care."

INA MAY GASKIN
Author, Spiritual Midwifery and Ina May's Guide to Childbirth

Feedback from Women Practicing Techniques from
Saving the Whole Woman

The following are posts taken from the forum on the Whole Woman™ website (www. wholewoman.com). They have been edited only for spelling and punctuation. These are just a small sample of results reported by hundreds of women from around the world.

This fire breathing is helping me. I want to sing it from the treetops. Thank you Christine!

GranolaMom

I have been to many doctors. None of them could figure out the pain, which was low abdominal, low back pain after bowel movements. I found this website and the posture information while researching, and within a few days of making posture corrections, the pain is mostly gone, AND my rectocele and cystocele have both gone from stage 2 to stage 1.

Tracy

For me, I will always be grateful for Christine, her materials, her inspiration and instruction, and for all of you who travel a similar path. By the way, the DVD exercises are still instrumental in my healing program. I didn't do them for a couple of days and I noticed!

Marie

I just turned 48 and had what I believe to be a global prolapse (cystocele, rectocele and uterine prolapse) happen all at once, within about a month or so around March of 2004. Thank goodness I found Christine's book and website!! I started using the posture immediately and I really believe it helped stop the progress of my prolapse.

Lynn

So I finally feel that my life is back on track with the discovery of your wonderful video and book. I thank God for giving me the help in finding you Christine.... and thank you so much!!!

Gail

I have to add that I JUST started doing the fire-breathing a couple days ago, and I think it is so amazing. I kept raving on and on to my husband! I was feeling a little 'droopy' on Saturday and so I gave it a go. I checked myself before, and could feel my cervix dropping to the middle of my vagina. I did the fire-breathing for 5 minutes and then checked myself again - IT HAD MOVED UP!!! Unbelievably (to me) it worked immediately! I never thought that was possible, although going for a long walk in the posture helps almost as much...eternal thanks, Christine.

MichelleK

I have come to the conclusion that standing in my 'old good' posture was just balancing the vertebrae on top of each other and not utilizing the muscles around the pelvis and spine to do the stabilizing, so all those muscles weakened and were unable to do the stabilizing work required when I was lifting. Now they get their strengthening exercise just by sitting, standing and walking. They are working all the time and much better for it.

Just remember that Whole Woman posture is at the heart of it. Just keep those pelvic organs forward of the pelvic floor opening and well over the pubic bone and they cannot descend because there is a big lump of bone in the way!!

Louise

I was told by my ob-gyn that I have UP [uterine prolapse] and adenomyosis and that a hysterectomy would be a "good option" for me. It was described as a procedure that could improve my quality of life. As a young-ish mother of two small children, wife, avid runner and outdoor enthusiast, I was devastated. My gut instinct told me that I had to research what surgery really meant, and find an alternative. I began researching surgical options...after reading those books, it is very easy to start feeling that your falling pelvic organs are the enemy and surgery is the key to restoring your quality of life. I was feeling a great deal of negativity toward my own body, as if there was something grossly wrong with me and I had been betrayed. I then read your book, and was reminded of what important parts of my body my pelvic organs are. Your book brought me back home...I feel so much more positive and confident that I have what it takes to work this out. I'm recommending it to my PT, sisters, and friends. Thanks so much for sharing your experience and research.

Thankful

Hi to all. I have been doing Christine's exercises for about a year. I have stage 3 prolapse, am 59 and always thought I was in pretty good shape. I have been feeling really good, so Sunday I decided to do some yoga and some abdominal work (my brain still tells me no pain no gain) to my surprise today my prolapse is back full force. So it's back to Christine's video and my abdominal tape went in the trash. As soon as I went back into the posture and relaxed a little I was feeling better. This is a way of life for me now and I believe it's not the worst thing that can happen to a woman. Thanks to all and a special thank you to Christine.

Rosemary

The Posture is working!

MommyNow

The posture has helped me no end - No longer do I have a falling out feeling or 'peeking'

Sue

I have also improved tremendously since I first found the prolapse a week post partum. My cervix, which was initially at the vaginal opening, has not re-prolapsed and although it is still a little lower than before I had children is now in a place which is considered "normal" for multiparous women and is causing no problems.

UKMummy

Christine's work saved me from surgery: cesarean section and pelvic surgery. I am so grateful for this work. I sit a lot on the floor because it is much easier to be in the posture and so much more comfortable than furniture. At work I tilt the front of my seat forward and do not even use the back rest. I have been increasing the nuts in my diet which has really caused the rectocele (the more troublesome of the three prolapses for me) to be no trouble.

I am so excited about Christine's new book and encouraged that doctors are finally listening. Perhaps in the future prolapse will be eradicated through our lifestyle changes as the medical community stops turning to the scalpel to correct a structural problem.

Jane

I just want to say that I am so, so very glad that I found your website all those three years ago.... I am still doing very well now. The posture has been a miracle worker.... I get it! It is now so natural to me to stand and sit in this posture... I can't even imagine putting myself back into the old stance, it seems it would be very difficult to even hold my body in that position anymore. As I said, in a few other long past entries, this posture not only brought everything up and secure and prevents any further prolapse no matter how much I lift or what I do physically. But more, it brought out my innate elegance, strength, self-confidence, beauty and power. Perhaps it was a grand combination of many changes colliding together in one synergistic point in my life, but what ever it was, I have grown to become, in many ways, a new person....or maybe it is that I found not a new person, but come nearer my real and truer, uncontaminated, God-blessed self.

Sandy-Joy

I just wanted to let you know I am already feeling better just from practicing the posture and getting down on all fours like you outlined in you post First Aid For Prolapse. I haven't even gotten my book yet, but I've ordered it and I can't wait. I am so, so thankful that I found this site when things are still relatively mild and can hopefully be reversed. I am believing that they will be! Already I have had several days where I do not even feel the bulging sensation. God bless you, Christine for your work here.

Julie

I am mindful of my posture and live by the rules that women with prolapse should follow (I've learned it all from this website). I hope to keep my prolapse where it is for a long while.

Marcella

Christine, I am very thankful and appreciate all of your hard-work, wonderful work, and all the precious information. There is a positive energy and you give women all the hope that they have lost in their own bodies. Thanks for saving us!

Anna

I was diagnosed with a 1.5 cystocele and a "slight" rectocele about a year ago. Last week, my gynecologist declared both "mostly resolved." I have had zero symptoms the last few weeks, but I also know that symptoms can come and go. Over all, things have improved hugely and continue to improve.

Ann

Saving
the
Whole Woman

ॐ

*Natural Alternatives
to Surgery for
Pelvic Organ Prolapse
and Urinary Incontinence*

Also by Christine Ann Kent

Diet for the Whole Woman–A Manual for Creating Total Health
First Aid for Prolapse DVD

Saving
the
Whole Woman

ഌ

Natural Alternatives
to Surgery for
Pelvic Organ Prolapse
and Urinary Incontinence

Christine Ann Kent

Illustrations by Nikelle Marie Gessner

Second Edition

BRIDGEWORKS
Albuquerque, NM USA

For the latest information on Christine Kent's work log on to: www.wholewoman.com.

ISBN   978-0-970-1440-1-0
ISBN   0-9701440-1-6

Library of Congress Cataloging-in-Publication Data

Kent, Christine Ann, 1952-
  Saving the whole woman : natural alternatives to surgery for pelvic organ prolapse and urinary incontinence / Christine Ann Kent ; illustrations by Nikelle Marie Gessner. -- 2nd ed.
      p. cm.
  Includes bibliographical references and index.
  ISBN-13: 978-0-9701440-1-0 (trade pbk.)
  ISBN-10: 0-9701440-1-6 (trade pbk.)
  1. Uterus--Prolapse--Alternative treatment--Popular works. 2. Pelvic floor--Diseases--Alternative treatment--Popular works. 3. Pelvic floor--Surgery--Risk factors--Popular works. I. Title.

  RG361.K46 2007
  618.1'45--dc22

2007031421

For educational or bulk purchase discounts, contact the publisher at the address below:

BRIDGEWORKS INC.
414 1/2 Central Ave SE, Suite 4
Albuquerque, NM 87102
1-888-514-1400
www.bridgeworks.com

Important Notice to Readers

ღ

Further Information and Support

The Whole Woman™ website is your source for the latest information on Christine Ann Kent's research, writings, forthcoming books, workshops, and speaking schedule. Included is a Community Forum where you will be able to learn from and share your experiences with other women.

By registering on her site you can be notified of her speaking schedule as well as be the first to receive announcements about forthcoming publications and workshops. Log on today at:

www.wholewoman.com

ღ

Classes and Personal Instruction

Christine Ann Kent's Whole Woman™ Center in Albuquerque, New Mexico, offers individual work with her and classes in The Whole Woman™ Workout. Christine's DVD, *First Aid for Prolapse,* and other helpful products for women with prolapse as well as class schedules and other Center information can be found at

www.wholewomancenter.com

ღ

For my mother, who never understood her agony

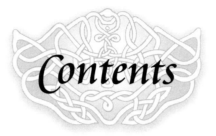

Contents

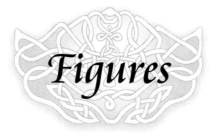

Figures

Acknowledgements

My sincere appreciation goes to all the women from the forum on the Whole Woman™ website (www.wholewoman. com). Your questions and sincere hunger for information have sent me back again and again to the medical literature. You have motivated me to keep digging deeper to solve the riddles of our anatomy, correct the misguided assumptions of the medical system, and learn how we can heal ourselves. In addition, your success stories, insights, friendship, and support to the forum have motivated me to keep moving forward even when the work felt overwhelming.

This work would not have been possible without the generous help of my family. My very talented daughter, Nikelle Gessner, provided endless revisions of the many technical drawings in the book. My brilliant son, Arien Gessner, developed the first iteration of the Whole Woman™ website. My loving husband, Lanny Goodman, has provided consistent design, technical, financial, and emotional support from this work's inception.

Bless you all!

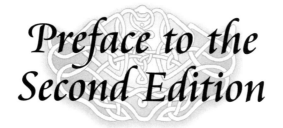

Preface to the Second Edition

It is said we all have a special purpose in life, a unique gift no one else can offer. I never believed it was true. But in the year 2000 during a health crisis I saw myself in a powerful vision: a woman I did not yet know, confident, smiling and doing her life's work. I called my mother to tell her I had "seen" that one day I would have a Center in Albuquerque where I would be teaching something of great importance. During the long silence that followed I could almost hear her eyes roll. Five years later I had traded my country life for the priceless gift of sharing my dharma at the Whole Woman™ Center.

I put the first edition of *Saving the Whole Woman* together during the two years after my vision and at times felt that the book was writing itself. What a thrill it was to receive validating endorsements from the top of my "wish list" of persons reviewing the manuscript.

In February 2004 wholewoman.com was launched and my son, Arien, at the time a budding Internet marketer, insisted that I include an online forum and "community of interest" on the site. No way could I see myself leading such an affair. However, no amount of protest could convince him of that, and, since he was building my website, up went the Whole Woman™ Forum.

Within 24 hours women began writing in to share their stories and inquire about this new alternative. I answered the first question, and the second, and the third, and thought to myself, "Surely I've told them everything I know." More and more women joined in, sometimes three and four a day, as something completely magical began to unfold.

The questions and topics presented seemed to roll out in an order that couldn't have been more enlightening had they been scripted. I kept responding, sometimes aided by medical literature and other times going back to the well of my own experience. I carefully described the Whole Woman™ Posture again and again and again.

Within weeks women began posting messages of elation and gratitude. They were getting results! Not just one woman, but dozens and dozens until I lost count. From the beginning I was very careful to state this was not a cure or quick fix, but rather a way to live well with prolapse by stabilizing and sometimes reversing symptoms. There was no question I had discovered a profound truth.

Even though in my book I had quoted a public health study, which stated that prolapse was not a disease of "little old ladies," I was not remotely prepared for the number of newly prolapsed, postpartum mothers desperately in search of information and support. Our blessed Jane, who goes by the user name "fullofgrace," showed up very early on in the life of wholewoman.com, pregnant with her third child and prolapsed since the birth of her second.

She quickly assimilated the concepts we were working with, adopted the Whole Woman™ Posture, and made the decision to have a gentle home birth. Her birth story, permanently posted on the website, serves as a beacon of hope to other pregnant mothers with prolapse. Over the following months and years my original theory of pregnancy and prolapse emerged, and is detailed in the Pregnancy & Prolapse chapter.

Readers of both books will notice that I did not include the historical chapter "Journeying" in this second edition. It was highly charged with emotion and horror, and although I believe it is very important that women connect the dots between our historical past and surgical present, many found it more disturbing than helpful. I have replaced that information with solid theories and evidence of why we should do everything in our power to preserve our natural design and leave the Age of Reconstructive Pelvic Surgery behind forever.

The concepts contained in these pages could not have been easily conveyed were it not for the almost 100 new and original anatomical illustrations created by my daughter, Nikelle. All have either been re-drawn from classic texts or based on current scientific understanding. With these we hope to enlighten and inspire you the reader, and also correct long-standing anatomical errors in the medical literature.

I tried my hardest to replicate the beginning posture and movement program just as it is being taught here at the Whole Woman™ Center. I hope you enjoy the companion CD, for although there is no short cut to re-building the musculoskeletal frame, there is also no more enjoyable way to do it than to beautiful, inspiring music. May you develop a love and desire for practice.

Christine Ann Kent
July 15, 2007
Albuquerque, New Mexico

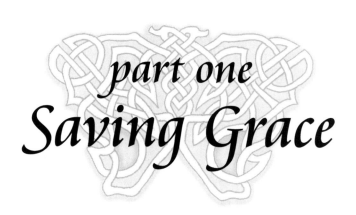

part one
Saving Grace

And the falcon is a pretty bird,
Wanders as she flies.
She asks us easy questions,
We tell her easy lies.

MIMI AND RICHARD FARIÑA[1]

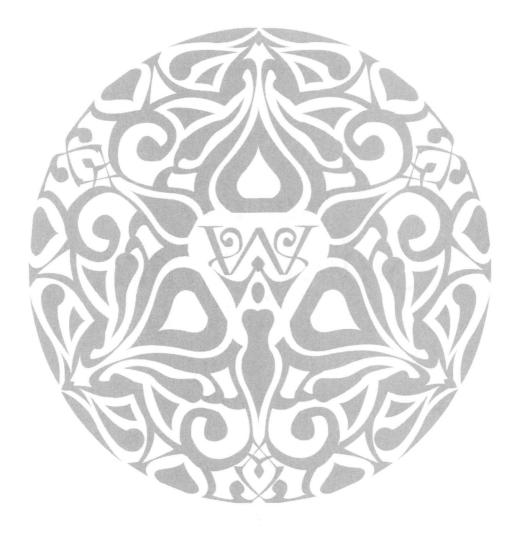

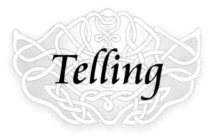

Telling

A Daughter of the world, whose Spirit was forged under pain and strife, has completed her spiritual raiment. She draws open the heavy curtain so that Light might pour forth, and summons the call to a new order of Reality.

STORYTELLING IS AT THE HEART of human existence. Our personal stories call into being dream, vision, and experience so that others may share in our knowledge of the world. The most powerful stories come from our collective experience, which reveals universal truths about darkness and light, connecting and holding us in unity. The story I am about to tell is at once glorious and grave. It is a story of the vital and perfect nature of woman, her descent into darkness and destruction, and her return to wholeness by the natural grace of flawless design. This is a story women have been waiting to be told for generations, and one we must continue to tell our daughters and their daughters throughout the world through all time.

We are going to see a culture divided from itself and dependent upon 3,000 years of abstract reasoning. We will learn that in the process of abstraction, reality has been restricted, severely limiting our ability to comprehend our place within the grand scheme of nature. We will understand how the two driving characteristics of Western culture, power and control, have shaped our medical system, and how women continue to suffer the brutality of dominionism in the name of "surgical correction," "cure," and "protection." We will come to know the high cost associated with dependence, disorientation, and loss of control, while discovering the equally great reward of restoring ourselves to health. Listen closely as I begin a story sure to rattle your bones, and follow me on a journey toward redefining reality, recreating health, and restoring sanity to a civilization that prompted Mahatma Gandhi to remark, "One only has to be patient, and it will be self-destroyed."[1]

The story begins with my own story, which had its beginning in the fall of 1993 when I was forty-one years old. During a routine pelvic examination, I was diagnosed with a large uterine fibroid and bluntly advised by my gynecologist that I needed a hysterectomy. Other than occasional episodes of leaking slight amounts of urine when I coughed or sneezed, I was experiencing no symptoms of pelvic difficulty whatsoever. Although it

was becoming common knowledge at the time that fibroid tumors are almost never ma-
lignant, are extremely prevalent in the industrialized world, are diet sensitive, and stop
growing at menopause, my doctor made my condition sound serious and suspicious as
she urged me toward consent. I quickly sought a second opinion and was told that, yes, a
hysterectomy was really the only reasonable option for me.

Although my mother and sister had been hysterectomized, and both tried to help
me see value in the operation, my instincts told me NO WAY. I called my trusted gynecologist from years earlier when I lived in another part of the country. He assured me the
fibroid could be removed by modern laser surgery and that there was probably no need
for hysterectomy. Relieved and resigned to the inevitable myomectomy (fibroid removal),
within a month I was on an airplane and in the hands of my doctor, a well-educated ob-
stetrician/gynecologist who practices medicine at one of the most prestigious hospitals in
Southern California.

After examining me and inquiring about any and all symptoms I was having, I told
him of my occasional episodes of mild urinary incontinence. He replied that I was "too
young for that kind of thing" and recommended I have my bladder "tucked up" as long as
he was "going to be in there anyway." I asked him to describe any and all risks, to which
he responded there were none, outside the usual surgical risks of anesthesia and infection,
and that there might be a slight change in the stream of my urine. It all sounded safe and
sensible to me. Little did I know that every part of my being had been enculturated to
mistrust my own judgment about the workings of my body and to trust completely in this
handsome, well-established man in the white coat.

We were scheduled for surgery the following day, which I was looking forward to as
a necessary, if aggravating, consequence of having a female body. After the usual surgical
preparation and total anesthesia, my pelvic cavity was accessed by laparotomy, a low incision just above the pubic bone. The fibroid, the size of a large egg, was removed using the
laser, and the wound in my uterus sewn closed with permanent sutures. The "tucking up"
of my bladder was accomplished via the Marshall-Marchetti-Krantz procedure—a major surgical operation where, after dissecting and tunneling down behind my pubic bone,
layer upon layer of skin, fat, connective tissue, nerve, lymph, and blood vessels, my bladder
and urethra were exposed and filled with blue dye for easier observation. The neck of my
bladder was re-angled and the connective tissue surrounding it securely sutured to the
muscle of my abdominal wall. My initial recovery was "uneventful," with the associated
nausea, vomiting, extreme pain, and tearing sensation as I retched for hours in reaction to
the anesthesia. A supra-pubic catheter (a small, firm tube that is inserted by puncturing all
the way through the abdominal wall, threading it toward the bladder, and then piercing it
directly into the bladder), used to evaluate the post-surgical flow of my urine, was found to
have a leak in the tubing, but luckily I did not develop an infection.

When the doctor and I agreed that I was strong enough to make the trip home, I traveled back on the airplane with plenty of pain medication on board and the abdominal dressing intact. A few weeks after the surgery I was feeling well enough to walk outside under the brilliant Indian summer sun. Walking back across the yard toward my house, I felt an odd sensation in my vagina, rather like something falling out. Not quite registering the experience, I walked slowly into the bathroom to investigate, only to encounter the large "something" bulging from my vagina. To say the least I was terrified to find an internal organ protruding from my body. In a panic, I called my California surgeon. With an affect of shock and disbelief he exclaimed, "How in the world did that happen?" I hightailed it to my local doctor who diagnosed a stage-three uterine prolapse. I called the surgeon back to tell him the news and he replied that unfortunately all surgeries to resuspend the uterus are completely unsuccessful and this was now a truly serious condition requiring hysterectomy.

I never spoke to the California physician again. Even with my rudimentary knowledge of pelvic anatomy and physiology, I knew the bladder surgery had caused my uterus to prolapse. I sent for my operative report and was outraged to see the long list of risks and complications (prolapse not among them) he stated to have discussed with me. He also stated that because of my "significant incontinence, the operative procedure was *first suggested by the patient*."†

I saw a total of four more gynecologists in an effort to gather as much information as possible about uterine prolapse. I was not interested in any more surgical "solutions," and three of the four doctors treated me as if I were out of my mind for thinking I could manage prolapse naturally for the rest of my life. I found it amazing that both male and female gynecologists had the very same conceptual framework, at best merely tolerating ideas and suggestions outside their area of expertise. In any event, I was fitted for a pessary (a rubbery diaphragm-like device to hold up prolapsed pelvic organs) and began learning and intuiting everything I could about naturalizing my pelvic organ support system.

My progress was slow and discouraging at first. Parts of my pubic area near the surface scar were (and still are) completely numb. Urination now required great effort. On the lower right side, deep into my pelvic cavity dwelled a constant, dull ache. My bowels behaved differently, and the glands above my pubic bone became swollen and sore with sexual activity, sex itself no longer working as it had before the surgery. Certain positions were very painful to maintain; it was as if my vagina had been repositioned. My menstrual periods also became very difficult. Where once menstruation was regular, relatively pain-free, and unobtrusive, now each month I had to deal with pain and heaviness in my abdomen, lower back, legs, and even the arches of my feet! Most discouraging was the big, boggy uterus bulging out between my legs.

Two years after the surgery, standing at the nurses station of the hospital where I worked as a registered nurse, one of our orthopedic surgeons approached me from behind and asked why my right scapula (shoulder blade) was "winging out so far." I replied that I

---

† *Emphasis mine*

wasn't aware it was, but further investigation revealed not only was my scapula protruding, but also my right shoulder and right hip were significantly higher than the left. This was certainly a recent development, as I had studied ballet during adolescence and throughout my twenties and knew quite well the condition of my strong, symmetrical body.

My body's deeper whisperings told me the surgery had also caused my entire musculoskeletal structure to be pulled grossly out of alignment. As symptoms usually are, my deep, throbbing, right-sided pelvic pain was a signal that something much more systemic was going on. There is an old Zen instruction, "Break your bones!" that teaches, "The Way is without difficulty. Strive hard!" More determined than ever to find non-invasive ways to neutralize the damage done to my body, I gave my body permission to teach me its awesome truth, while I proceeded to break old, calcified patterns of thought and conditioning. So began the healing journey at the heart of our story through hushed medical libraries, dusty archives, ribald women's circles, and skilled therapeutics, urged forth by a cacophony of ancient, insistent female voices.

∞

Pelvic Organ Support

Science is not a fruit of the spirit of truth, and this is obvious as soon as one looks into the matter.

Simone Weil
The Need for Roots [1]

LONG AGO, WHEN OUR ANCESTORS lived in the great forests of the Old World, tree branches held the weight of their agile bodies as they went about all their activities of daily living. Their extremely nimble hands revealed to them their world as they reached for thousands of varieties of green leaves and colorful fruit, groomed their loved ones, and traveled about their homeland. If they wanted to sit they would prop themselves up on their hands and wrap their sturdy tail around their base, much like a cat.

We began to learn that if we balanced our body in this sitting position, our hands were completely free and our voice box stabilized and supported. Our legs, crossed and folded beneath us, provided a broader base than our tail had given, so we traded our tail for sturdy sit bones and large, heavy buttock muscles upon which we could comfortably sit. From this seated posture our whole universe lay before us. Our spine straightened and our brain grew as we turned our gaze toward the heavens and began to contemplate the brilliant night sky (Figure 2-1).

Intra-abdominal pressure, coming down from our lungs every time we take a breath, is the "force" that allowed us to fix our body in this position, giving us the ability to rotate our head, use the full range of our voice, and work with our hands.[2]

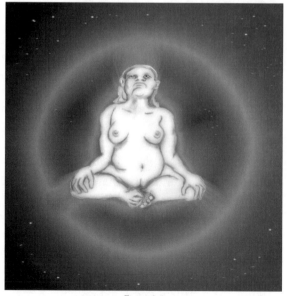

Figure 2-1

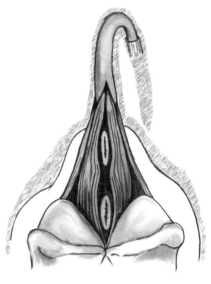

Figure 2-2
Caudalis Muscles

When we desired to use our two legs to stand for longer periods and to cover greater distances, the human female had to overcome a unique design problem. How would we remain upright and withstand not only gravity, but also the tremendous intra-abdominal pressures generated while talking, walking, running, jumping, lifting, coughing, laughing, sneezing, and still be able to give birth to large-headed offspring without our pelvic organs falling out the bottom?

Four-legged creatures solve the problem of intra-abdominal pressure by remaining on all fours. In this posture their pubic bones serve as a strong osseous shelf above which their pelvic organs are positioned. It is the pubic bones that form the floor of the quadrupedal pelvis. At right angle to the bony animal pelvic floor is a group of muscles called the caudalis muscles. The pubocaudalis, iliocaudalis, ischiocaudalis, and sacrocaudalis muscles form a strong vertical wall surrounding the pelvic outlet and pelvic sphincters. It is the separation, or genital hiatus, down the entire length of the caudalis muscles through which the animal urethra, vagina, and anus open to the outside of the body (Figure 2-2). Contraction of the caudalis pelvic diaphragm helps to equalize abdominopelvic pressure and maintain control of the pelvic sphincters. However, the main role of this strong vertical wall of muscle is to wag the animal tail in all directions. Intra-abdominal pressure, as well as pressure from a full bladder and rectum, is exerted against the abdominal wall in quadrupeds and not against the pelvic sphincters. Therefore, danger of pelvic organ prolapse and urinary and fecal incontinence is minimal.[3]

Occasionally, four-legged mammals desire to stand on two legs. When they attempt to do so their pelvic organs exert direct pressure upon their pelvic orifices. Consequent-

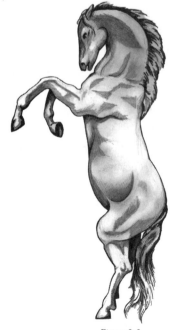

Figure 2-3

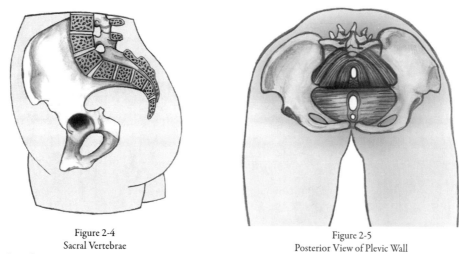

Figure 2-4
Sacral Vertebrae

Figure 2-5
Posterior View of Plevic Wall

ly, risks of spontaneous evacuation and organ prolapse greatly increase. Animals standing on two legs cope with pressure increases by strongly contracting their caudalis muscles and drawing their tail sharply underneath between their hind legs. In this way, brief periods of time standing on two legs can be tolerated without developing incontinence or prolapse (Figure 2-3).[4]

As we will later learn, for hundreds of years scientific medicine believed that in order to accomplish bipedalism the human pelvis rotated backward around the hip joints to become a basin-like structure with the pelvic diaphragm as a horizontal "floor" at the bottom.

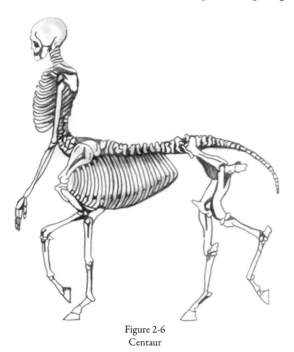

Figure 2-6
Centaur

However, we now understand the human pelvic diaphragm remains more vertically oriented than that of the quadruped. When we stood up it was our lumbosacral spine that allowed us to do so by bending sharply from horizontal to vertical. Our first three sacral vertebrae are horizontal (Figure 2-4). Our pelvis remained in the same position as all other four footed animals, while the rest of our body stood upright[5] (Figure 2-5). The mythological centaur best illustrates the true relationship between our pelvis and abdomen (Figure 2-6).

Pelvic organ support is the acquired result of normal human ac-

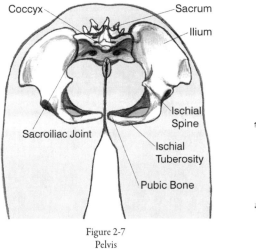

Figure 2-7
Pelvis

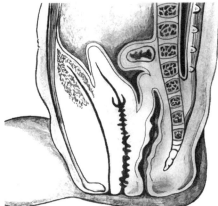
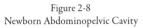

Figure 2-8
Newborn Abdominopelvic Cavity

tivity. Arising from wave forms generated by our breath above and our feet striking the ground below, a central ring of support develops to harness, balance, and direct the essential energy of human movement. The osseous pelvic ring is composed of three bones and six moveable joints (Figure 2-7). The sacrum is the large triangular bone at the base of our spine made up of five fused vertebrae for maximum stability. Two-to-four tiny fused bones below our sacrum form our coccyx, or tailbone. On either side of our sacrum are two wing-shaped hipbones, or ilia, which connect to either side of the sacrum through

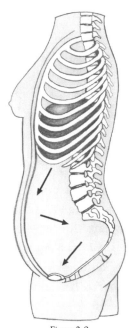

Figure 2-9
Intra-abdominal Pressure

the sacroiliac joint. At the back of the ilia are two deep circular depressions into which fit our femurs, or thighbones. Behind these are the ischial tuberosities or bony protuberances we know as our sit bones. The ilia in front and ischia in back meet to form the two flat, horizontal surfaces of the pubic bones. These come together like the straps of a saddle underneath our torso and between our legs and are connected by a fibrous disc called the symphysis pubis. The cylindrical birth canal has both an *inlet* at the ilia and an *outlet* at the tailbone.

Energy created in our lungs every time we take a breath moves through our torso in a very specific pathway and actually creates the shape of the female body. The newborn abdominopelvic cavity is one long, funnel-shaped space (Figure 2-8). Infant organs are protected from prolapse because both the thoracic diaphragm underneath a baby's lungs, and her pelvic diaphragm, are made up of the same type and same amount of muscle tissue, so internal pressures simply bounce back and forth between the two sets of muscles. It is only through standing, walking, running and jumping that intra-abdominal pressure begins to exert its full effect upon the shape of the female body. [6] The respiratory diaphragm grows thick and strong and begins sending powerful bursts of energy through the torso.

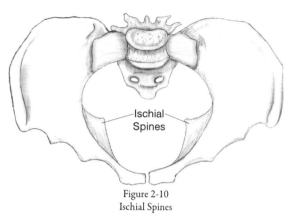

Figure 2-10
Ischial Spines

Over the course of childhood and adolescence energy thrusts from above move the bladder and uterus, which are carried high in the newborn abdomen, into the pelvis. The downward and backward movement of pressure (Figure 2-9) creates tension in our spine and causes the pelvic diaphragm to pull forward on the lower sacrum and coccyx, curving these structures and tightening the area between the ischial spines. The ischial spines, which are almost nonexistent in tailed animals, become strong bony protuberances in the human that turn inward at the level of the mid-pelvis and onto which insert many important muscles and connective supports for the urethra, vagina, and rectum (Figure 2-10). In natural standing posture, traction is increased upon the ischial spines and the pelvic diaphragm is tightened across its diameter.

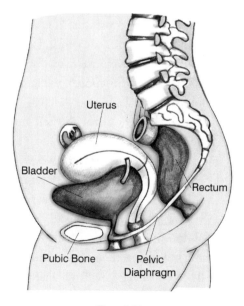

Figure 2-11
Pelvic Anatomy

This movement results in greater angulation of the spinal column, which creates the pronounced female lumbar curve. By late puberty the relentless forces of intra-abdominal pressure have been pushing the pelvic contents down and back from the abdominal wall.[7] Evidence of this process can be interpreted from the geometry of the pelvic interior. The marked lumbosacral angle defines the positions of the organs under pressure, keeping the bladder, uterus, and sigmoid colon locked into place near the lower abdominal wall instead of being forced toward the pelvic outlet (Figure 2-11).

Unlike animals taking erect posture, in which case internal forces are transmitted totally to the pelvic diaphragm, the acquired shape of the female spine prevents intra-abdominal pressure from being transmitted directly to the pelvic outlet. This is because the abdomen and pelvis are no longer in line with one another, or no longer have the same *axis* (Figure 2-12). The mature human female abdomen and pelvis end up at right angles to one another, resulting in the pelvic organs becoming biaxial as well. By the end of puberty, the axis of the urethra forms an almost right angle with the bladder, the vagina with the uterus, and the rectum with the sigmoid colon. These natural folds act as passive sphincters in what has been called the "autoblocking mechanism" of pelvic organ support. In standing posture the vagina flattens to an airless space and remains unaffected by the forces of internal pressures. Intra-abdominal pressure is first exerted upon the uterus, accentuating its anteflexion, or forward positioning. As a consequence, the uterus is pushed over the bladder dome, which in turn is pushed down and foward over the pubic bone. Pressure is transmitted through the bladder to the vesicovaginal septum, or space separating the bladder and vagina. Because of

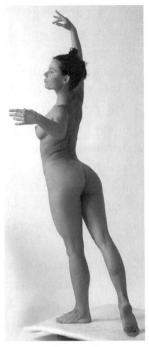

Figure 2-12

the flattened vagina, it moves directly to the rectovaginal septum separating vagina and rectum, and on to the perineal body of the pelvic diaphragm. The tone of the pelvic interior increases in response to intra-abdominal pressure, making the vaginal angle more acute: the greater the pressure, the more acute the angle (figure 2-13). This geometry of the biaxial pelvis prevents the vagina from folding back upon itself under pressure.[8]

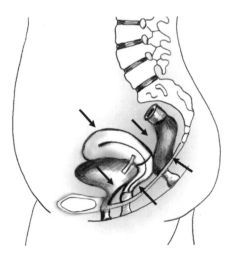

Figure 2-13
Increased Angles with Increased Intra-abdominal Pressure

Intra-abdominal pressure coming down from our lungs every time we take a breath creates both form and function of the female pelvic organ support system. Babies and young children breathe through their nose as their lower abdomen rises with inspiration and falls with expiration. However, by adulthood most people in the developed world have reversed the process and actually breathe backwards! They do this by pulling in their abdominal muscles with inspiration while using muscles in their upper chest and neck to lift their ribcage. Such a maladapted breathing pattern not only creates tension and musculoskeletal discomfort, but slowly

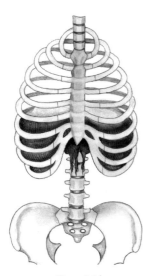

Figure 2-14
Respiratory Diaphragm

dislodges the pelvic organs from their natural positions.

Breath is flowing through our body every moment we live. Yet, it is only when we become fully upright that the breath, under tremendous pressure from gravity, literally sculpts our natural form. Movement of air into and out of our lungs is accomplished by the major and accessory muscles of inspiration and expiration. When we breathe in, or inspire, we use the respiratory diaphragm and external intercostal muscles. The respiratory diaphragm is a dome-shaped muscle separating the heart and lungs above from the abdominal cavity below (Figure 2-14). Lining the entire inner circumference of the chest wall, the diaphragm is attached to the inner surfaces of the lower three pairs of ribs and strong bands of connective tissue arising from the lumbar vertebrae. When the diaphragm contracts downward it increases the volume of the chest cavity and creates a vacuum that draws air into the lungs. [9]

During natural inspiration the abdominal wall stretches out anteriorly (forward) while the abdominal and pelvic contents are pressed down and forward over the pubic bone. The abdominal muscles must be relaxed for natural breathing to occur. The combined movements of the muscles of inspiration and the abdominal wall pull the lumbar spine forward, reinforce the lumbosacral angle, and pin the pelvic organs into normal anatomic positions.

During exhalation the diaphragm relaxes upward in a passive recoil movement that requires no muscular effort. When breathing out, the internal intercostal muscles that travel at right angles to the external layer, gently pull the ribs down and inward. The abdominal muscles come more into play during deep and forced exhalations when they contract to lift and hollow the abdominal cavity. The deepest set of abdominals, the transverse abdominis, act like a girdle around the lower belly and are gently exercised as they pull in with each exhalation. The shallow breathing that occurs when the abdominal muscles are constantly pulled toward the spine reduces the tone and condition of the transverse abdominis. The deeper the breath is pushed into the lower belly, the more these muscles are conditioned. The transverse muscles also act to stabilize the abdominal wall when they are lengthened on the inhalation.

The breath flows from an area of the body that must remain both rigid and flexible. The chest must be strong enough to protect the heart and lungs, as well as provide attachments for many powerful muscles throughout the torso. Yet, this area must also remain flexible in order to function as a bellows during the inspiration/expiration cycle. Rigidity and points of muscle attachment are provided by the bony ribcage and shoulder girdle. The pliability that also characterizes the rib cage results from the ribs being separate from one another and attached to the sternum by flexible cartilage. Resilient attachments to spinal vertebrae also provide significant mobility. The entire structure of the ribcage provides continuous elastic tension so when it is stretched by muscle contraction during inspiration it can recoil passively to resting dimensions when the muscles relax.

Our breath becomes an intra-abdominal force as soon as the diaphragm contracts downward. With each inhalation the abdominal and pelvic organs are massaged down and forward as the abdominal wall expands. Peristalsis, or the movement of food through the digestive system, is dependent upon the rise and fall of our breath. The pelvic organs are affected by inspiration in exactly the same way, as evidenced by their horizontal, forward placement within the pelvis.

The human body is two-thirds water and the movement of intra-abdominal pressure through the aqueous environment of the inner pelvis is much like that of a tidal pool ebbing and flowing in continuous wave forms. Just as ocean waves carve a coastline, patterns of energy moving through the pelvis create both the form and function of pelvic organ support. Continuous thrusting of the lower bowel against the hollow of the sacrum distends the pelvis toward the back. With each natural inhalation, the respiratory diaphragm descends by pulling forward on the lumbar spine. In this way angulation of the spine at the lumbosacral junction increases, lumbar curvature expands, the inner aspect of the sacrum becomes markedly concave, and the tailbone curves toward the pubic bone as tension increases across the width of the pelvic wall.

Opposite waves of energy spiral up from the ground with every step we take. The great muscles of our legs and buttocks increase the intensity of compressive forces generated at the foot-ground surface. The upward-moving energy, filtered and shaped by elastic structures within our knee, hip, and sacrum, becomes perfectly harmonious with the downward-moving spiral created by our breath.

The ascending energy is sequentially delivered to the collagenous disc between each spinal vertebra. This results in compression and rotation of the intervertebral joint. The lumbar vertebrae, already drawn forward by traction from the respiratory diaphragm, bend sideways with the compressive force. Lateral rotation of the lumbar spine results in a high level of torque that drives one side of the pelvis forward. This is the biomechanical process we use to walk and run.[10]

The upward-moving energy spiral repeats this process for each intervertebral joint, and upon reaching the thoracic spine, counter-rotates the shoulders. After shoulder rotation, the energy spiral moves on to the cervical spine. The axial torque created by the shoulder movement would cause the head to wobble were it not for the unique shape and arrangement of the cervical vertebrae. These change the dynamics of the energy wave, reversing the direction of torque and canceling out any remaining energy at the top of our spine so that our head remains stable.[11]

At the center of these spiraling waves of energy is the architectural ring of power upon which pelvic organ support depends. The pelvic ring is the hub of a wheel of muscle, ligament, and the tough, fibrous connective tissue known as fascia that unites the trunk above with the extremities below. Natural female posture "winds up" the pelvic ring so that the whole body moves into a geometry of greater stability.

The mechanism of the self-locking pelvis is centered at the sacroiliac joints and supported by the mass action of muscle, fascia and ligament throughout the rest of the body. Before we take a closer look at the anatomy of the self-locking pelvic ring, let us define certain concepts and terminology that aid in describing our three-dimensional body as it moves through space.

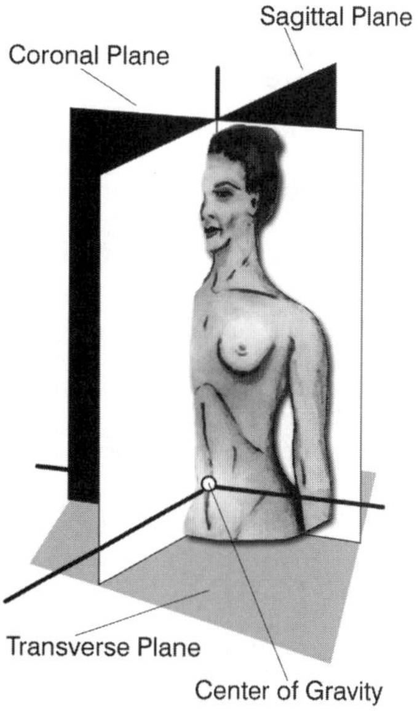

Figure 2-15
Anatomical Symmetry

Planes, Axes, & Center Of Gravity

Planes, axes, and center of gravity are geometric terms for describing body position and movement. Planes describe dimension and divide the body front-to-back, side-to-side, and top-to-bottom. The sagittal plane intersects the body equally by weight into right and left halves. The coronal plane intersects the body equally by weight between front and back halves. And the transverse plane divides the body equally by weight between top and bottom.

An *axis* is a line drawn between the intersection of two body planes. A line formed from the intersection of the sagittal and coronal planes measures height and is called the *vertical axis*. A line formed from the intersection of the coronal and transverse planes measures width and is called the horizontal axis. A line formed from the sagittal and transverse planes measures depth and is called the anterior-posterior axis. The intersection of these three body planes creates a point. This point is the center of gravity from which all movement and stability derive (Figure 2-15).

Anterior & Posterior

Anterior and posterior designate front and back.

- The anterior vaginal wall is near the urethra.
- The posterior vaginal wall is near the rectum.

Proximal & Distal

These terms describe a body part or portion of an organ as near or far from the trunk or base point.

- The proximal urethra is at the bladder opening.
- The distal urethra is near the opening where urine exits the body.

Medial & Lateral

These describe a movement or body part as near or far from the midline of the body.

- Your navel is medial to your hip.
- Your arm is lateral to your spine.

Ipsilateral & Contralateral

These describe the same or opposite side of the body.

- Your right arm is ipsilateral to your right leg.
- Your right arm is contralateral to your left leg.

Abduction & Adduction

Movements away from and toward the body are described by the terms abduction and adduction. Abduction is a movement away from the body in the coronal plane. Adduction is movement toward the body in the coronal plane.

- The leg is abducted when lifted out to the side.
- The leg is adducted when lowered back toward the body.

Flexion & Extension

Muscle stretching and shortening produce basic body movements known as flexion and extension. Flexion is a bending, or closing movement, while extension is a straightening, or opening movement. Examples of flexion and extension are as follows:

- The hip is flexed when the leg is raised to the front
- The hip is extended when the leg is raised to the back.
- The lumbar spine is flexed when the tailbone is tucked under and the lumbar curve flattened.
- The lumbar spine is extended when the tailbone is lifted and the lumbar curve present.

Nutation & Counternutation

When the pelvic ring is loaded with weight from above, as when we sit up straight

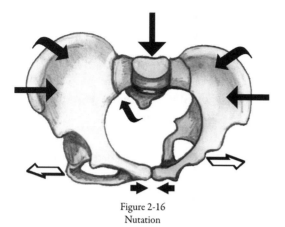

Figure 2-16
Nutation

or stand, the sacrum moves into the self-locking position that winds up, or tightens, the soft tissue structures of pelvic organ support. When we sit back or slouch, the sacrum moves out of its locked position as surrounding tissues slacken. This back and forth rocking motion at the sacroiliac joints is described as either nutation or counternutation.

Nutation occurs when the top of the sacrum moves down and forward toward the interior of the pelvis, and the tailbone lifts up and back. The iliac crests, or tops of the hipbones, move down and medially, while the ischial tuberosities, or sit bones, spread apart. The front of the symphysis pubis squeezes together while the back of the symphysis widens (Figure 2-16). These are all very slight movements, yet because they are at the hub, or center of the body, have far-reaching effects. Sacral nutation is responsible for crucial elements of pelvic organ support:

- Nutation is initiated by the in-breath, which causes the respiratory diaphragm to pull forward on the lumbar spine.

- Nutation increases the lumbar curve at the base of the spine, which stabilizes the pelvic organs near the lower abdominal wall where they are pinned into place by the forces of intra-abdominal pressure.

- Nutation causes the pelvic wall to lengthen from pubic bone to coccyx, and to tighten across the ischial spines.

- Nutation causes the deep perineal muscle to tighten, which stabilizes the urethra and vagina.

Counternutation occurs when the top of the sacrum moves up and back from the pelvic cavity as the tailbone tucks under the rest of the spine. The iliac crests move up and laterally, while the ischial tuberosities move toward one another (Figure 2-17).

- Counternutation causes the lumbar curve to flatten.

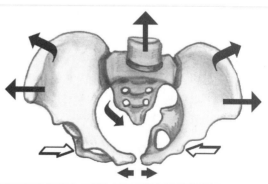

Figure 2-17
Counternutation

- Counternutation causes the pelvic diaphragm to shorten from pubic bone to tailbone, and to slacken across the middle as tension on the ischial spines is released.

- Counternutation slackens tension in the muscles surrounding and supporting the urethra and vagina.

In standing and seated postures, the pelvis is most stable when nutated. In this position the sacroilliac joints are locked into place by the shape of their bones and the strength of their ligaments. Sacral nutation creates the conditions for pelvic organ support. When the pelvis is nutated, the lumbar curve is present, the pelvic wall stretched along its natural axes, and the pelvic organs held forward over the pubic symphysis. During walking and running, the highly flexible pelvis alternates side-to-side between nutation and counternutation. The weight bearing side of the pelvis is nutated, while the contralateral side is loosened for the flexibility necessary to swing the opposite leg forward.[12]

How Muscles Work

Muscles that produce movement in the body are called voluntary, or skeletal muscle. Arranged in layers, muscles are described as either superficial or deep. Superficial muscles are nearest to the skin. Muscles consist of microscopic groups of fibers wrapped in envelops of fascia and bundled together into groups. These groups are further bundled together, enfolded in more fascia, and fastened with tendon at either end to a structural support, such as bone. Muscles work in groups simultaneously across joints to produce movement.

Muscles move bones by contracting, or sliding along their fiber bundles to shorten. Although able to stretch to one and a half times their resting length, it is through shortening of their fibers that muscles do their work. Muscles can only pull, they cannot push. The muscles doing the work of contracting, or pulling, are referred to as *agonists*. On the other side of the joint are found a different muscle group, the *antagonists*, which stretch and resist their counterparts. The same muscle can act as agonist or antagonist by either shortening or lengthening its fibers. Muscles can also increase their length under tension by keeping some of their fibers contracted, therefore acting as stabilizers instead of movers. Such is the case with the muscles of the pelvic diaphram.

Muscle tone refers to the responsiveness of muscle while in its resting state. Muscles with good tone respond instantly to nerve stimuli and effortlessly maintain posture. Muscle tone is involuntary, which means it cannot be consciously controlled. Our overall state of physical and emotional health determines our muscle tone. Tone is a concept that can be applied to connective tissue as well.

The Structures Of Pelvic Organ Support

Structures as far away as the base of our skull and soles of our feet join together in creating the architecture of pelvic organ support. Because mind and body work together, deeper understanding of structural organ support can only enhance the physical effort of restoring the beauty, grace, and function of our original design. The following is a brief study of some of the principal players in the self-locking ring of postural pelvic support.

Arches of the Foot

The foot is composed of three arches:

- The *transverse arch* spanning the medial-to-lateral margins of the forefoot.
- The *lateral longitudinal arch*, which spans the lateral portion of the foot from heel to little toe.
- The *medial longitudinal arch*, which spans the medial portion of the foot, from heel to big toe.

With each step, elastic energy is stored in the arches of the foot. This energy is then rebounded throughout muscle and fascia from the foot to the lumbar spine. This spring action helps to relieve some of the burden of lifting our leg from our core abdominal muscles.

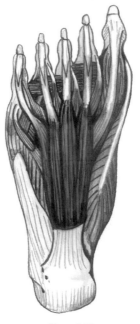

Figure 2-18
Foot Arch

Largely because of shoes and poor postures, many people in the developed world exhibit a flatness of the arches, angularity of the ankles and unlevelness of the sacral base. The natural human foot is wide and triangular with well-developed arches. Exercises that strengthen the arches and make them more flexible are essential to reestablishing proper function of the pelvic organ support system (Figure 2-18).

Thoracolumbar Fascia

The multi-layered thoracolumbar fascia (TCF) forms a deep tissue core around the bones and muscles of our spine and pelvis (Figure 2-19). Tone of the thoracolumbar fascia affects the stability of the female pelvic organ support system and is conditioned by the several muscles that connect to it, including the transverse abdominis, gluteus maximus and erector spinae. Whole body, weight-bearing exercise is required to properly tone the thoracolumbar fascia.

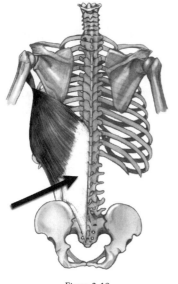

Figure 2-19
Thorocolumbar Fascia

Erector Spinae

Three sets of deep spinal muscles run along either side of the vertebrae from sacrum to skull. As their name implies, the erector spinae serve to lift, or extend, the spine into the vertical position (Figure 2-20). Through broad attachments to the sacrum, the erectors pull forward at the lumbosacral junction, inducing nutation. During side bending they flex the trunk laterally.

In Whole Woman™ Posture, the erector spinae enhance the lumbar curve and limit the thoracic curve. They do this by maintaining a state of mild contraction. Chronic, insufficient nutation of the sacrum weakens the erectors and limits their normal role as antagonists to the pelvic diaphragm and muscles of the abdominal wall.

Quadratus Lumborum

This flat muscle at the front of the spine reaches between the upper back rim of the pelvis and the lowest "floating" rib (Figure 2-21). Quadratus lumborum controls the connection between the back of the rib cage and the back of the pelvis and stabilizes the

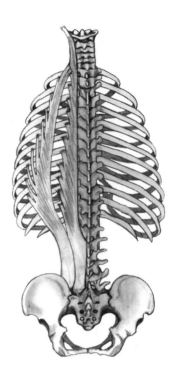

Figure 2-20
Erector Spinae

pelvis on the lumbar spine, therefore playing a major role in postural alignment.

Tightness in the quadratus lumborum combined with weak abdominal muscles can cause hyperextension, or swayback, in the lower spine. Quadratus lumborum is strengthened during exercises that rotate the trunk. During standing leg lifts, quadratus lumborum keeps the pelvis level and prevents collapsing onto the supporting leg. When standing in the Whole Woman™ Posture, quadratus lumborum acts with the erector spinae to extend the lumbar spine.

Iliopsoas

Although often referred to as simply "the psoas," the iliopsoas are really two different muscles with distinct functions that unite to

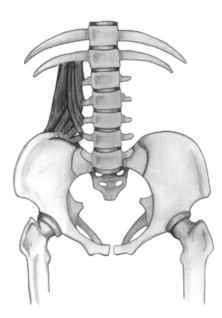

Figure 2-21
Quadratus Lumborum

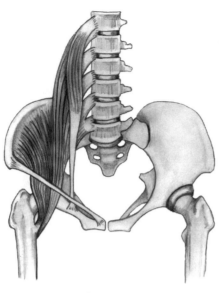

Figure 2-22
Iliopsoas

form a common tendon, which inserts onto the top of the femur (Figure 2-22). The flat, broad iliacus muscles line the inside of the ilia and extend from the iliac crests and sacroilliac joints to the top of the femurs. Contracting across the hip joint from iliac crest to femur, the iliacus pulls the pelvis forward on the hip joint to create a forward bend. The iliacus muscles are continuously active during walking and running and are strengthened with standing leg lifts.

The psoas muscles originate on the sides of the lower thoracic and lumbar vertebrae, course down and laterally through the pelvis in front of the hip joint, and join the iliacus to insert onto the femur. The psoas connects the lower back with the legs and is a powerful stabilizer and flexor of the hip joint. During a standing leg lift to the front, psoas is strengthened. When the outstretched leg is carried to the side and back, this muscle is lengthened.

Standing postures that pull in the abdominal muscles and tuck the pelvis weaken the ability of the psoas to stabilize the lumbar spine. Tight, weak psoas muscles are accompanied by flexion at the hips, resulting in misalignment throughout the pelvis and spine. The Whole Woman™ Posture lifts the upper body from deep in the pelvis, lengthens and strengthens the psoas, and correctly aligns the legs with the torso.

Gluteus Maximus

These powerful hip extensors also serve to abduct and rotate the thighs laterally (Figure 2-23). Gluteus maximus originates on the back of the ilium, sacrum, and coccyx and has two insertion points, one on the femur and the other on the lower leg. It is gluteus maximus contracting that allows a standing leg lift to the back. Because of the double insertion points, it plays a role in both abduction and adduction of the thigh. A powerful lateral rotator of the thigh, gluteus maximus acts as a prime mover and stabilizer of the legs and trunk during all

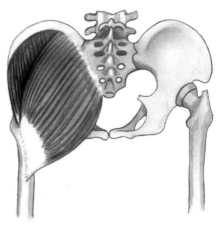

Figure 2-23
Gluteus Maximus

upright activity. Contracting the gluteals in standing posture pulls the spine into flexion and disrupts pelvic alignment. Tight psoas muscles in front and weak gluteals behind lead to the major postural deformity associated with loss of pelvic organ support.

The Hamstrings

The three muscles arising from the area of the sit bones and coursing down the entire length of the back of the thighs are known as the hamstrings. The medial hamstrings run down the inside of the thigh and insert below the knee. These work to rotate the extended thigh inward. The lateral hamstring is the prime mover known as biceps femoris (Figure 2-24). In concert with the gluteals, this muscle lifts and rotates the thigh to the back. These are the muscles that flex the knee and when tight prevent the thigh muscles from fully stretching the knee joint. This in turn limits flexion at the hip.

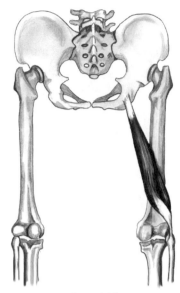

Figure 2-24
Biceps Femoris

By way of their ligamentous attachments to the pelvis, these muscles work as antagonists to the muscles that extend the lumbar spine. Short hamstrings limit forward bending, induce counternutation of the sacrum, and flatten the lumbar curve.

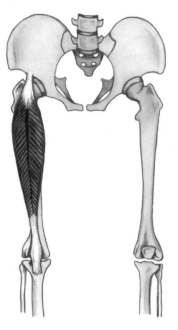

Figure 2-25
Quadriceps Femoris

Quadriceps Femoris

Four separate muscles at the front of the thigh make up "the quads". The largest of this group, rectus femoris, attaches proximally onto the front edge of the ilium near the hip joint and distally below the knee (Figure 2-25). The main function of the quads is to extend the knee, but because rectus femoris originates at the hip joint it is also a powerful flexor of the hip. If there is weakness in the psoas muscles, which are the primary hip flexors, rectus femoris will take over this action. The anterior thighs then become bulky and overworked, resulting in loss of strength and efficiency of the hamstrings. The Whole Woman™ Posture lengthens and strengthens the core psoas muscles, which in turn balance the muscles of the thigh.

The Adductors

The five muscles in the adductor group arise from the anterior and posterior aspects of the pubic bone (Figure 2-26). Pectineus is the only adductor that attaches to the anterior aspect of the pubic bone, while adductor longus, adductor brevis, gracillis, and adductor magnus arise from the posterior aspect. The point of origin of adductor magnus is posterior to the pubic symphysis and all the way to the ischial tuberosity. Adductor magnus and adductor longus attach to the back of the femur while gracillis attaches below the knee. The adductor muscles draw the legs toward each other and rotate the thighs medially acting as antagonists to the gluteal muscles to stabilize the legs during all upright activity. Different insertion points cause some of the adductors to also act as lateral rotators of the thigh. Sitting in a right-angle posture with the lumbar curve in place while medially rotating outstretched legs maximally lifts the urethra into its functional position.

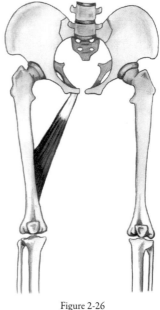

Figure 2-26
Adductor Longus

Deep Lateral Rotators

The deep outward rotators of the thigh are quadratus femoris, obturator internus, obturator externus, piriformis, gemellus superior, and gemellus inferior (Figure 2-27).

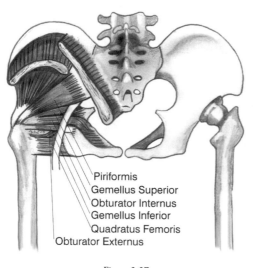

Piriformis
Gemellus Superior
Obturator Internus
Gemellus Inferior
Quadratus Femoris
Obturator Externus

Figure 2-27
Deep Lateral Rotators

These six small muscles underneath gluteus maximus act as important stabilizers of the hip during walking. Arising from different points around the sacrum and lower pelvis, they pass out of the pelvis behind the hip joint to attach onto the great knob, or trochanter, of the femur. These muscles rotate the thigh laterally in the non-weight-bearing leg and abduct it when sitting. It is the deep outward rotators working when you move your leg to the side to get up out of a car seat. (See page 25 to learn more about the relationship between obturator internus

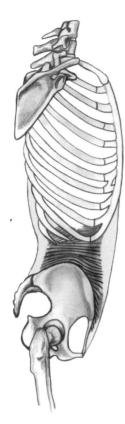

Figure 2-28
Transverse Abdominis

and pelvic organ support.)

The deep outward rotators are stretched to their functional length in Whole Woman™ Posture.

The Abdominals

Rectus abdominis, the external obliques, internal obliques and transverses abdominis form a corset-like network around the front of the torso. The most superficial layer, rectus abdominis, run vertically on either side of the abdominal midline from pubic bone to sternum and function primarily as spinal flexors. Rectus abdominis mirrors the action of the pelvic diaphragm. The middle abdominal layers are the internal and external obliques, which assist in rotation of the spine and lateral bending of the trunk. They also help replace the abdominal organs under the respiratory diaphragm during expiration.

Transverses abdominis are the deepest of these muscles, which course horizontally around the abdominal wall from back to front (Figure 2-28). These are the muscles that pull the abdominal wall toward the spine during passive and forced exhalation. The transverses abdominis also hold a mild contraction during natural female posture so the belly can be relaxed, yet supported.

Latissimus Dorsi

These great muscles of the back originate from the iliac crests, sacrum, lumbar vertebrae and lower six thoracic vertebrae (Figure 2-29). They branch out laterally to connect with the lower ribs, then course under the scapulae before inserting onto the long bone of the upper arms. The way the head, arms and shoulders are held in seated and standing postures has a tremendous effect on the function of the lower spine and pelvis. Likewise, the way the pelvis is positioned on the lower extremities affects the comfort, strength, and flexibility of the upper body.

The latissimus dorsi is the muscle that connects the arms directly with the lower back and pelvis.

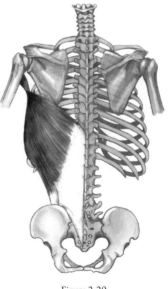

Figure 2-29
Latissimus Dorsi

Reaching around the scapula and underneath the armpits, it assists the muscles of the upper back in stabilizing the shoulder girdle and rotating the arms. This muscle is a prime mover of energy across the sacroilliac joint and works with the contralateral gluteus maximus to compress and stabilize the sacrum in nutation.

Trapezius

The shoulder girdle is formed by the sternum and collar bones, or clavicles, in front and the shoulder blades, or scapulae, in back (Figure 2-30). Unlike the massive, ligament-wrapped pelvic ring, the free-hanging shoulder girdle has but one bony connection to the rest of the trunk. In this way the rib cage is allowed maximum mobility for respiratory function.

The trapezius muscles act almost exclusively to rotate, elevate, depress, abduct, and adduct the scapulae. Arising near the base of the skull and upper vertebrae, the trapezius drapes like a shawl over the

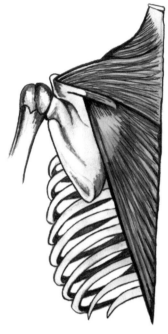

Figure 2-30
Trapesius

shoulders and attaches onto the scapula and back of the clavicle. In the Whole Woman™ Posture, it is the muscle most responsible for holding the shoulders down. Trapezius also contracts to allow arching of the head and upper back.

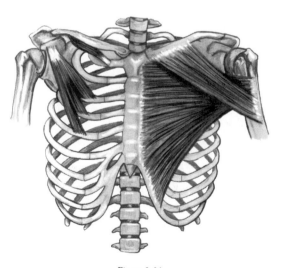

Figure 2-31
Pectoralis Muscles

Pectoralis Muscles

These large muscles of the chest act as both prime movers and stabilizers of the arms and shoulders (Figure 2-31). Pectoralis major arises from the clavicle, upper ribs and sternum. It then travels toward the shoulder to insert onto the long bone of the upper arm. These muscles assume a major role in adducting the arms and when the arms are raised above horizontal they depress the clavicle and keep the shoulder girdle pulled down.

The deeper pectoralis minor

arises on the upper ribs and attaches to the scapula. By pulling forward on the shoulder blades, this muscle has a primary role of lifting the rib cage. Pectoralis minor works antagonistically with trapezius by pulling the shoulders forward while trapezius pulls them back. Balance between these two sets of muscles is important. Habitually slouched posture causes the pectoralis muscles to become shortened and weak, which manifests as chronically rounded shoulders and inability to stand up straight.

Deltoid

This muscle capping our upper arm and shoulder connects to the clavicle in front and the scapula in back before inserting onto the long bone of the arm (Figure 2-32). These extensive connections allow the deltoid to move the arm in all directions. Acting with the pectoralis muscles the deltoid pulls the arm forward. With the latissimus

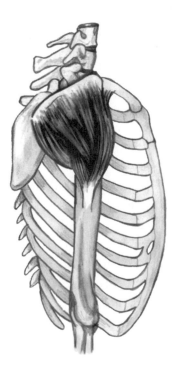

Figure 2-32
Deltoid

dorsi it draws the arm to the back. The deltoid functions as prime mover in abduction of the arm and as an accessory muscle in all other arm movements. The Whole Woman™ Posture positions the shoulder girdle correctly and minimizes workload on the deltoid. Consequently, the shoulder does not become overly bulky in proportion to the rest of the arm.

Sternocleidomastoid

As its name implies, this strong, thick muscle on either side of the neck originates on the upper portion of the sternum, the upper border of the clavicle, and inserts into the bony protuberance behind the ear known as the mastoid process (Figure 2-33). These muscles bend the head laterally toward the

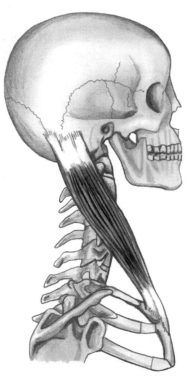

Figure 2-33
Sternocleidomastoid

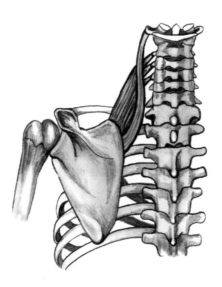

Figure 2-34
Levator Scapulae

ipsilateral shoulder. They also rotate the head and turn the face upward to look toward the contralateral side. When both muscles contract, the head and neck are brought forward into flexion. Turning the head to the side before bending the upper spine backward allows the sternocleidomastoid muscle to hold a controlled, elongated contraction in order to support the structures of the head and neck.

Levator Scapulae

Located at the sides of the neck and underneath the upper trapezius, these narrow, strap-like muscles originate on the cervical vertebrae and insert onto the upper borders of the scapulae (Figure 2-34). The levator scapulae lift and rotate the upper edges of the scapulae. In the Whole Woman™ Posture, these are the muscles that stretch the neck upward as the shoulders are kept down.

Muscles of the Pelvic Outlet

The levator ani and coccygeous muscles, together with their fascial coverings, enclose the opening at the back of the pelvis. The levator ani is formed by the pubococcygeus muscles and the iliococcygeus muscles (Figure 2-35).

The pubococcygeus muscles arise from the anterior aspect of the pubic bones and from the levator branch of the arcus tendineus (Figure 2-36). The arcus tendineus is a fibrous structure that runs across the middle of the pelvic sidewall from the ischial spine to the pubic bone. This important anatomical structure allows for separate functioning of muscle groups of the pelvic outlet. As it nears the pubic bone, the arcus branches out into a Y shape. The lateral arm of the Y becomes the arcus tendineus levator ani and the medial arm the arcus tendineus fascia pelvis. In this way the muscle action that controls the back of the pelvic outlet can be separated from the fine motor control of the urinary system.

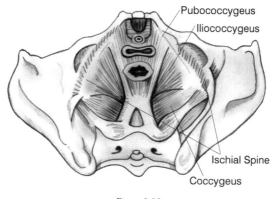

Pubococcygeus
Iliococcygeus
Ischial Spine
Coccygeus

Figure 2-35
Pelvic Wall in Lithotomy Position

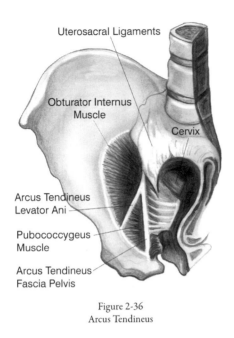

Figure 2-36
Arcus Tendineus

Obturator internus shares this common attachment site with the levator ani muscles. Habitual standing and walking with turned out feet shortens and weakens both sets of muscles, favors counternutation of the sacrum, instability at the sacroilliac joint, and pelvic organ prolapse.

The puboccygeus blends in the midline with the outer vaginal walls and perineal body before inserting into the front and sides of the coccyx. The iliococcygeus surrounds the pubococcygeus and fuses behind the rectum. The coccygeus muscles extend from the tailbone to the ischial spines. Embedded in these muscles are the sacrospinous ligaments, which stabilize the full extension of the pelvic wall. In the Whole Woman™ Posture, the muscles of the pelvic outlet are lengthened from pubis to tailbone and made taut across the middle by tension between the ischial spines.

The Urogenital Diaphragm

Two layers of muscle form a strong and supportive shield across the front half of the pelvic outlet below the levator ani (Figure 2-37). The urogenital diaphragm is a muscular triangle that runs across the diameter of the pubococcygeus and attaches along the front and sides of the pubic bones. Both layers are covered by deep fascia on their superior and inferior surfaces. The superficial layer contains muscles that surround, stabilize, and compress the vaginal opening and clitoris. The deep layer contains the deep transverse perineal muscle. This important muscle is part of a muscular network known as the external urethral sphincter because of its role in maintaining the urinary continence system.[13] The deep transverse perineal muscle wraps around the distal portion of the urethra, envelops the vaginal opening, and then fans out laterally to form a muscular triangle across the anterior half of the pelvic outlet (Figure 2-38).

When the sacrum is fully nutated, the front of the pubic sym-

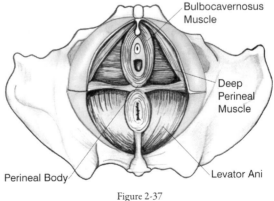

Figure 2-37
Urogenital Diaphragm in the Lithotomy Position

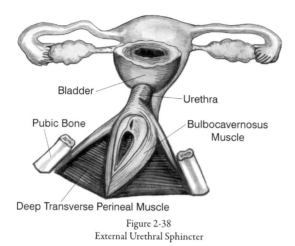

Bladder

Urethra

Pubic Bone

Bulbocavernosus
Muscle

Deep Transverse Perineal Muscle

Figure 2-38
External Urethral Sphincter

physis is compressed due to its close proximity to the ilia, which are also compressing medially. However, nutation causes the ischial tuberosities to move away from one another laterally, resulting in decompression, or widening, at the back of the symphysis. The ischiopubic rami, or portion of the pelvis between the symphysis and ischial tuberosities, widens with nutation. As the sit bones move apart, the urogenital diaphragm tightens across the middle, elevating and stabilizing the urethra within its muscular framework.

The perineal body is a major support structure often referred to as the central tendon of the pelvis. Between vagina and anus, this pyramid-shaped, fibromuscular structure connects across the pelvic outlet to either side of the ischiopubic rami by way of the deep transverse perineal muscle. The perineal body is indirectly attached to the tailbone by the external anal sphincter, which is attached at its other end to the coccyx. The perineal body serves as an anchor for soft tissue structures of the perineum, yet its fiberous core also provides the distensibility necessary to rebound against intra-abdominal pressure.[14]

Generations of women are living today with the long-term effects of episiotomy, which can result in the perineal body slowly disintegrating, the back vaginal wall becoming directly exposed to intra-abdominal pressure, extreme thinning of tissue at the back of the introitus, or vaginal opening, and pelvic organ instability.

Endopelvic Fascia

Most gynecologic surgeons who contribute to peer-reviewed literature agree that actual "ligaments" do not exist within the pelvis. Rather, the same tough, stretchy fascia that envelops each organ and muscle extends from these structures to connect onto the walls of the bony pelvis. The endopelvic fascia (Figure 2-39) is the major support structure of the pelvis and the primary reason disorders of organ support cannot be compartmentalized, but rather must be considered as a whole.

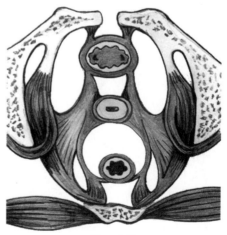

Figure 2-39
Endopelvic Fascia

Nerves of the Pelvic Wall

Because nerves move muscle, proper electrical supply is necessary for normal functioning of the pelvic organ support system. The deep levator ani muscles receive direct nerve stimulation from the second, third, and fourth sacral nerves of the lower spinal cord (Figure 2-40). A separate conduit called the pudendal nerve arises from this same sacral plexus and travels to the back of the pelvic wall where it stimulates the perineum. The pudendal nerve has three branches: the clitoral branch that travels along the perineal membrane to supply the clitoris; the perineal branch that supplies the perineal muscles; and the hemorrhoidal branch that supplies the external anal sphincter muscle. Nerves run alongside the blood vessels throughout the pelvic wall. The pudendal nerve and its branches play a central role in the innervation of the anal and urethral sphincters, thus maintaining urinary and fecal continence. Laboratory analysis of pubococcygeus tissue reveals a combination of slow twitch (type I) and fast twitch (type II) muscle fibers. A predominance of type I fibers suggests that the primary role of this muscle is to provide static structural support. However, the significant percentage of type II fibers present in the pubococcygeus indicates that it also helps to narrow and compress the genital hiatus.[15]

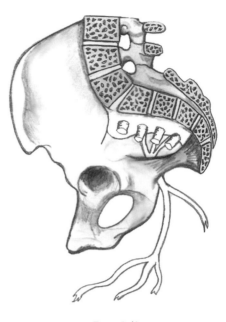

Figure 2-40
Nerves of the Pelvic Wall

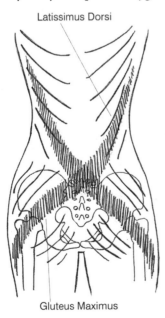

Latissimus Dorsi

Gluteus Maximus

Figure 2-41
External Compression of Sacroiliac Joint

Pelvic Organ Support

Pelvic organ support is a product of sacral nutation and the mass action of muscle, ligament, and fascia surrounding the bony pelvic ring. When the pelvis is loaded with weight from above, as with upright posture, the top of the sacrum rocks forward into the pelvis as the tailbone lifts up. The iliac crests move medially and down to wedge the sacrum into position. The gluteus maximus and latissimus dorsi muscles contract on opposite sides of the pelvis creating a bilateral compressive force across the sacroilliac joints and reinforcing nutation (Figure 2-41).[16] The pubic symphysis is compressed in front and widened in back. The muscles of the pelvic wall are stretched to their functional length from pubis to coccyx, producing tension on the coccygeal muscles in which the sacrospinous ligaments are embedded and tightening the pelvic wall lengthwise. This tension increases traction on the ischial spines and tightens the pelvic diaphragm across the middle. The posterior aspect of the symphysis and ischiopubic rami, or area of the pelvis in between the pubic bones and sit bones, widen, rendering the urogenital diaphragm taut. Like snapping open an umbrella, the fully extended urogenital diaphragm stabilizes the support structures of the urethra and vaginal opening.

If the breath is allowed its natural course, the lumbar vertebrae are pulled forward with inspiration and the pelvic organs pushed toward the lower abdominal wall. In this position the organs are compressed and pinned into place by pressure from the downward-moving respiratory diaphragm.

The evolution of the female pelvic organ support system is an exquisite story of how nature used the limiting forces of stress and gravity to create our fully human capacity to stand, walk, run, and leap—sometimes while singing and holding an infant. As you will see next, many things in our modern lives cause this magnificent design to weaken and collapse. However, the sacred way in which bone, muscle, ligament, fascia, and vessels are woven together into a seamless whole allows for a lifetime of enjoying our full human potential as well as the grace of regaining that capacity by returning to the original form and function of our natural design.

∾

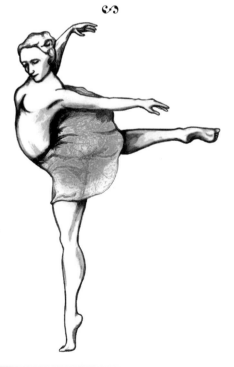

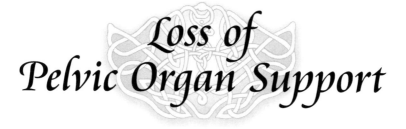

Loss of Pelvic Organ Support

Too much leisure and luxury can destroy our natural beauty as much as too little of life's necessities. Harmony and grace are born from the marriage of plenty and poverty.

GYÖRGY DOCZI
The Power of Limits[1]

*A*N ELEGANTLY DESIGNED female pelvic organ support system allowed us to keep the advantages of our "hind quarters" (sitting, squatting, climbing, running, easy elimination, easy birthing), while freeing the full use of our hands, voice, vision, and height.

Millions of years of evolution granted us a system capable of dramatic change during childbirth and subsequent return to pre-pregnancy proportions and function. Primatologists tell us that the shape of the human pelvis emerged 3.5 million years ago. They also describe one of the most unique features in all of evolution, the fact that a very large portion of life span of the human female is lived after menopause. The current theory states that older females have always benefited the human community (primarily by caring for older children while daughters were busy with newborns), therefore making our success as a species possible.[2] This could not have occurred if females had inherently weak pelvic tissues and pelvic organs susceptible to disease.

In the domesticated woman, however, many factors contribute to the now common condition of loss of pelvic organ support. As the greater skeletal framework around the organs changes, abnormal tension on pelvic soft tissue supports is increased. This stretching of ligaments, combined with breaks and separations in the endopelvic fascia, lead to a gradual or sometimes sudden fall of the bladder, rectum, small bowel, or uterus into the vaginal canal. The terms cystocele, rectocele, enterocele, uterine prolapse, and vaginal vault prolapse have been traditionally used to describe the bulging of various pelvic organs into and out of the vagina. Stress urinary incontinence (SUI) is the common experience of losing small amounts of urine during activities that sharply raise intra-abdominal pressure, such as coughing, sneezing, running and jumping.

Cystocele occurs when the bladder falls from its original position behind the lower abdominal wall and presses against the front wall of the vagina (Figure 3-1). In severe cases, the vaginal wall bulges outside the introitus.

Prolapse is commonly described by stages. At Stage 1 the organs are slightly displaced; at Stage 2 they are at or near the introitus; and at Stage 3 protruding beyond the vaginal opening. Stage 4 is a fully everted vaginal prolapse, an extremely rare occurance in the un-hysterectomized woman.

As we learned in the previous chapter, the primary difference between a woman's backbone and that of a four-legged creature is in how her spine and pelvis develop during her first years of life. Consistent standing, walking, running, and jumping cause her

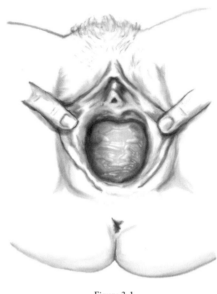

Figure 3-1
Cystocele

lower spine to form a great arch over her pelvic organs. Natural spinal development creates this uniquely human anatomy whereby her bottom half remains as horizontal as four-legged animals, while her chest, arms, shoulders, and head become fully upright.

Because of developmental differences between the sexes, the female spine forms an even more pronounced lumbar curvature than the male (Figure 3-2), creating the possibility for a perfect balance that keeps her pelvic organs positioned horizontally in the hollow of her lower belly like quadrupeds, but allows the freedom and grace of fully upright movement.

Traditionally in medicine, prolapse of the front vaginal wall has been described as

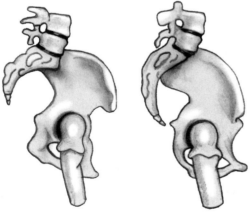

Figure 3-2

Female Pelvis   Male Pelvis

either urethrocele, or cystocele. Urethrocele may appear as a small bulge in the lower third of the front vaginal wall. In theory the support structures binding the urethra to the pubic bone have relaxed, allowing backward rotation of the urethra. This condition is referred to as urethral hypermobility and is often associated with stress urinary incontinence.[3]

When the normal urethra is well supported behind the pubic

bone, its upper portion lies above the pelvic wall. In this position it is within the pelvic boundaries that are subject to intra-abdominal pressure. Activities and movement that cause sudden pressure increases result in both the bladder and urethra being compressed equally (Figure 3-3A). Because the diameter of the normal urethra is so much narrower than that of the bladder, urethral pressure is greater than bladder pressure at rest, remains so during activity, and no incontinence occurs. When the urethra falls backward away from the pubic bone, the portion that was once within pelvic boundaries is now outside the forces of intra-abdominal pressure (Figure 3-3B). With stress activity like running, coughing, or sneezing, pressure is exerted on the bladder as before, but the urethra remains beyond the intra-abdominal pressure realm. Pressure inside the urethra is no longer increased by abdominopelvic forces and the resting pressure within the urethra is not enough to equal that being applied intra-abdominally to the bladder.[4] The result is stress urinary incontinence. Although the pathophysiology of stress urinary incontinence has been debated for over a century, it is generally accepted that if the support structures of the urethra slacken, stress urinary incontinence results despite otherwise normal urethra and bladder anatomy.

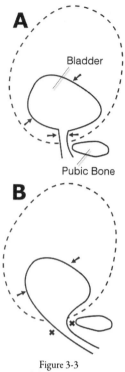

Figure 3-3
Intra-abdominal Pressure on
Bladder & Urethra

Cystocele is further classified into two sub-types, (1) distention cystocele and (2) displacement cystocele. A distention cystocele is also commonly referred to as a central defect and believed to result from overstretching of the front vaginal wall beyond its ability to involute, or normalize, postpartum. A distention cystocele presents as a smooth bulge in the front vaginal wall and is also considered to be a normal part of aging (Figure 3-4).[5] However, young women who have never given birth are also known to develop classic distention-type cystocele.

A displacement cystocele is thought to be a stretching or separation of the vaginal sidewalls from their attachments to the fascial coverings of the obturator internus muscles. Theoretically, this separation can be either unilateral or bilateral and is said to often create a combination urethrocystocele. Since the va-

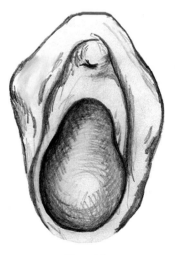

Figure 3-4
Distension Cystocele

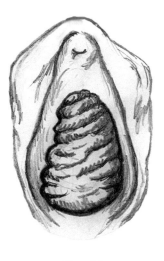

Figure 3-5
Displacement Cystocele

gina is attached to the pubocervical fascia at the pelvic sidewalls, a break in this area is thought to cause the sides of the vagina near the cervix to descend, the urethra to become hypermobile, and stress urinary incontinence to manifest. A diagnosis of displacement cystocele is made when the natural folds, or rugae that allow the vaginal walls their full expansion at childbirth, are present (Figure 3-5).

An adult female bladder filled with urine is a heavy organ poised within a cavity created by a spine that has managed to both remain horizontal and become vertical. The bladder is tucked well into the horizontal portion of the female body, but is not immune to forces that might pull it back toward the pelvic outlet (Figure 3-6).

It is well known amongst pelvic surgeons that collapse of the front vaginal wall does not often exist in isolation.[6] Rectocele is the bulging of the rectum against the back wall of the vagina and into the vaginal canal (Figure 3-7). The vaginal wall itself is often considered to be the defective agent in rectocele, however, this is a misconception because it is actually a chronic situation where alterations in intra-abdominal pressure cause the rectum to press against and stretch the back vaginal wall. As the vaginal wall gives way, the rectal wall has more leeway to balloon anteriorly, which causes the vaginal wall to become stretched even more. A combination cystocele/rectocele is the most common presentation of pelvic organ prolapse.

Urogynecologist and author Linda Brubaker highlights several studies showing 1st, 2nd, and 3rd degree rectoceles present in asymptomatic women—women who had no idea they had a diagnosable condition until they were examined in blind studies. She states, "It is certain that some anterior rectal wall movement is normal during straining, but the point at which this movement should be considered abnormal has not been established."[7]

Women become symptomatic when they begin to feel heaviness and a dragging sensa-

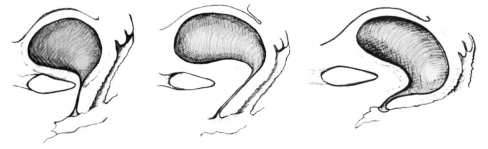

Figure 3-6
Progressive Cystocele

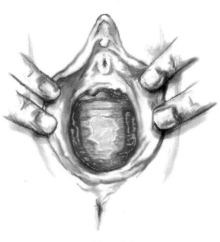

Figure 3-7
Rectocele

tion in the anal area, when feces trapped in the rectal bulge requires manual evacuation, and when they experience aching or pressure after a bowel movement. Compression of the rectum by the herniated sac may create the sensation of fullness even when the rectum is empty. Rectoceles can affect sexuality because of discomfort from large protrusions or loss of retained feces during intercourse.

In normal anatomy the vagina flattens to an airless space. If the vagina is being held slightly open by a developing cystocele or uterine prolapse, intra-abdominal pressure is exerted abnormally against the vaginal walls. It is very common for women to develop rectocele soon after or concurrently with cystocele. Straining against the toilet seat is a primary risk factor for all these conditions. Traditionally, rectoceles have been categorized as low, mid-vaginal, or high depending upon their presentation at the back vaginal wall. However, more careful observation has revealed that naturally occuring rectoceles usually present low in the vagina, whereas rectoceles recurring after surgical repair occur higher in the vagina or at the perineum.[8]

Descent of the perineum may or may not coexist with rectocele. Obstetric laceration, overstretching, or surgical revision can virtually obliterate the perineal body so that the lower posterior vaginal wall becomes exposed to inordinate levels of intra-abdominal pressure and forms what surgeons describe as pseudorectocele or *perineocele*. Upon examination however, the rectum demonstrates no abnormal bulging or irregular distension of the anterior rectal wall.[9]

Enterocele occurs when a section of small bowel sags into the space between the rectum and back vaginal wall (Figure 3-8). Just above this space, at the margin between the pelvic cavity and the intestinal cavity, the intestinal track curves slightly downward to form a small pouch of peritoneum, or sac that encases the bowel. This is known as the cul-de-sac of Douglas. A slight enterocele

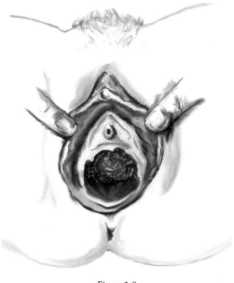

Figure 3-8
Enterocele

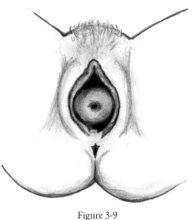

Figure 3-9
Uterine Prolapse

often accompanies uterine prolapse because the front wall of the cul-de-sac is connected to and drawn down along side the descending cervix. This is the very common "traction" type enterocele that is usually not diagnosed as a separate condition. The cervix helps to prevent a full blown entrapment of the small bowel between the back vaginal wall and rectum, which is a true enterocele. Symptoms such as feeling like the bowels are empty after a bowel movement only to have to sit back down a minute later as stool transit time is lengthened due to a deeper cul-de-sac are very common. A naturally occurring enterocele is seldom seen except in cases of birth defect or severe pelvic collapse. For three-quarters of a century, enterocele has been a well-known and extremely common post-operative complication of pelvic reconstructive surgery.

Uterine prolapse is the descent of the cervix or the entire uterus into the vaginal canal (Figure 3-9). Normally, the cervix is pointed slightly downward into the vagina and back toward the tailbone. The uterus bends toward the front of the body to rest its large base on top of the bladder. In this position, intra-abdominal pressure falls on the top of the uterus closest to the pubic bone, helping to keep it in proper position. If the pelvic support system weakens, the fascial and ligamentous network stretches and allows the cervix to move forward into the vagina.

In severe cases, the uterus turns the vagina inside out as it falls completely through and protrudes from the vaginal opening. However, because the lower part of the vagina is so well supported (it is the upper vagina that is very mobile) the cervix in most cases never descends more than a centimeter or so beyond the vaginal opening. Because the bladder and cervix are connected at the supravaginal septum they will always move in tandem. This means if the uterus is significantly prolapsed, the bladder will also be pulled well away from its normal position near the lower abdominal wall.

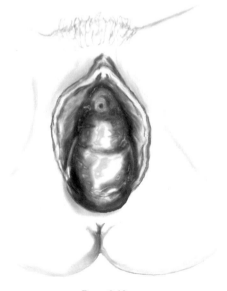

Figure 3-10
Vaginal Vault Prolapse

Vaginal vault prolapse occurs frequently after hysterectomy as the unsupported vagina itself turns inside out and falls through the introitus (Figure 3-10). This condition is reported to occur in up to 43 percent of hysterectomized women and requires further surgical intervention to permanently stitch the ballooned vagina back into the pelvic cavity.[10]

Loss of pelvic organ support is extremely common, affecting approximately 50 percent of women who have given birth in the developed world, and resulting in well over half a million surgical procedures performed annually in the United States.[11] There is an almost equal ratio of younger women to older women with symptomatic pelvic organ prolapse, and over the next thirty years we can expect a 45 percent increase in these disorders.[12] In postmenopausal women, 60 percent of gynecological surgeries are performed in an effort to correct dysfunctions of pelvic organ support.[13] Prolapse of the pelvic organs is the most common reason for hysterectomy in women older than fifty years of age. One study from Quebec found prolapse to be the reason for 13 percent of hysterectomies in all age groups.[14] Childbirth, straining on the toilet, connective tissue disorders, poor posture and pelvic surgery have all been correlated with collapse of female pelvic organ support.[15-20]

Childbirth is by far the greatest inciting factor, and we will see that it is obstetric or "instrumental" childbirth that is most suspect for having created an epidemic of pelvic support problems amongst Western women. Chronic constipation and straining to move the bowels has been observed to be more common in women who develop prolapse (61 percent) or stress urinary incontinence (30 percent) than in women who are asymptomatic (4 percent).[21] Connective tissue disorders (often a result of inadequate vitamin C and other elemental nutrients) and abnormal posture contribute to the fundamental cause of loss of pelvic organ support—the shifting of intra-abdominal pressure from the way it was directed during our evolution and development to a number of pathological courses.

Our pelvic organs are positioned in the pelvic cavity in such a way that intra-abdominal pressure keeps them in place and allows for proper functioning. As you are about to learn, all pelvic reconstructive surgery grossly disrupts these natural dynamics. When the surgeon tells you after prolapse or incontinence surgery not to lift more than a few pounds ever again, it is not because you may pull out stitches or strain a muscle. It is because he/she has completely altered the natural design of your pelvic system and anything you do, even standing and breathing, will now cause abnormal intra-abdominal forces to be directed in unnatural ways throughout the pelvic interior, often leading to further dysfunction.

Disorders of the pelvic organ support have been recorded for thousands of years. The first reports are from the Ebers papyrus, dating from 1500 B.C., which encouraged Egyptian women to smear their prolapsed uterus with honey and push it back into position. Hippocrates wrote in 400 B.C. that a prolapsed uterus should be sponged with cold wine and fitted with a pessary made of half a wine-soaked pomegranate. Cleopatra also proposed douching with astringent solutions in cases of vaginal prolapse.[22]

Loss of pelvic organ support is as old as civilization, and there is evidence that indeed it is a disorder of civilization. Two revealing studies have helped shed light on this fact. Thirty years ago the disorders of genital prolapse and urinary incontinence were rarely seen in Chinese women of Hong Kong. Since 1975 the territory of Hong Kong has undergone vast socioeconomic and demographic changes in order to resemble the industrialized cultures of the West. Greater material wealth has brought many changes, including Western medical practices and diets based more on processed fats and simple carbohydrates than traditional fiber-rich vegetables and grains. A 1975 study concluded that genital prolapse and urinary incontinence were rarely seen in Chinese women. By 1993, a second study of the same area found these conditions to be a significant portion of the caseload of most hospitals in Hong Kong.[23]

We have come to the dark and treacherous part of our story. It is not a story about the evils of all surgery or a condemnation of all pelvic surgeons. Surgery is a necessary, ancient, heroic art and many of its practitioners are highly sensitive, caring people. My own gynecologist is reputed to be the best pelvic surgeon in New Mexico and is a kind, gentle man who genuinely cares about women. Surgery is nothing less than miraculous when performed in cases of birth defect, trauma, gross pathology, malignancy, rupture, or elective procedures when the woman is made fully aware of all risks and benefits.

Rather, our story has as its central theme the rampant progeny of a century-old surgical furor: huge volumes of unnecessary, unsuccessful, and extremely damaging pelvic reconstructive surgeries born of the marriage between blind, rational thought and grotesque violation of women. The emperor of our story has no clothes. Pelvic reconstructive surgery is not even scientific! As you will soon discover, virtually no studies exist to prove or disprove its effectiveness. Yet, gynecologists and urogynecologists know exactly what they are doing when they perform over a million of these operations each year (not including the most common pelvic surgery—episiotomy) on American women. The problem was beautifully and artfully laid out in their own literature in 1934 and again in 1954.[24,25] Since then volumes have been published in the medical literature describing the intricate beauty of the female pelvic system and the copious problems faced trying to approximate that design with surgery. Yet, "Surgery has almost become the only widely available treatment for genital prolapse. Resident training in non-surgical modalities has almost disappeared,"[26] so that now up to 15 percent of American women seek surgical correction for loss of pelvic organ support during their lifetime.[27]

The social process of scientific medicine including absolute power, arcane language, ancient fraternity, and utmost loyalty, has blinded our doctors to some of the most basic truths of the female body. We catch a glimpse of the furor in the following quotation from a recently published pelvic surgery textbook: "Historically in gynecology, the treatment of urinary incontinence and pelvic organ prolapse was a pursuit occurring late in a physician's career. This observation gave rise to the saying, 'The obstetrician-gynecologist spends the first half of his career by supporting the perineum [episiotomy]and the second half of his career *being supported by*† the perineum.' More recently, a cadre of younger gynecologists has been able to concentrate on [profit from] the evaluation and care of patients with pelvic floor disorders, as have physicians in other disciplines, such as urology, general surgery, and colon and rectal surgery."[28]

The dynamics of the female pelvic organ support system are unique in the human body. Although pelvic surgeons often refer to prolapsed pelvic organs as "hernias," they are not. A hernia is a section of abdominal viscera that has burst through the musculature of the abdominal wall. These conditions are not subject to the same gravitational forces that prolapsed pelvic organs are and respond very well to surgical repair.

The twenty-first century is witness to an almost complete severance of women from both the knowledge of their bodies and their body of knowledge, which once kept them disease-free into old age. The medical establishment, over the course of several centuries, usurped female body knowledge from pubescent girls, mothers, midwives, healers, and menopausal women. Detailed technical knowledge has allowed gynecology to become very effective at solving complicated and rare female pelvic disorders. However, this in no way offsets the incredible harm done by the use of that same technology for common, benign conditions of the pelvis.

The next part of our story is difficult to read, as it was difficult to write. Nowhere in the public domain is there graphic, descriptive literature about what is done to the female body during pelvic reconstructive surgery. We are given appallingly patronizing terms like "tucks," "tie-ups," and "repairs," lulled into the death-sleep of anesthesia, and to awake astonishingly and incomprehensibly altered.

Some women return to their doctors again and again with infuriating and intractable symptoms until they are given the final referral—to the psychiatrist's office. Others recognize an old, familiar trap and choose instead to live with painful consequences, their heads down but somehow wiser. Walk with me through the dark and hellish tunnel. There is light at the end. It is the ancient, inextinguishable light of healing and protection shining forth from deep within our very bones.

ငဒ

---

† *Emphasis in original*

Surgical Intervention

Doctors never like being told that what they are doing is actually causing harm to their patients.

Te Linde's Operative Gynecology[1]

DOCTORS WHO PERFORM SURGERY for pelvic organ prolapse must share a unique cognitive dissonance. While they often proclaim prolapse to be a debilitating and irreversible condition for which surgery is the only cure, what they know is that their "cure" creates immense disability of which their profession rarely speaks. Enjoying ample and predictable revenues, gynecologists and urogynecologists must teach each other the delicate art of doublespeak as they ply the dual nature of their trade.

The classic textbook *TeLinde's Operative Gynecology* is the most revered, utilized, fundamental tutorial that exists on pelvic surgery. From this text we learn that, historically, all surgeries for pelvic organ prolapse that have preserved the uterus were utter failures so that today "Vaginal hysterectomy [removal of the uterus] has achieved a prime position in the treatment of mild and moderate degrees of symptomatic prolapse of the uterus."[2]

Struggling with the logic of their operative protocol, the surgeons continue,

In considering surgery for the correction of uterovaginal and other pelvic organ prolapse, the gynecologic surgeon is well advised to think of the surgical principles rather than just about a particular operative technique. For example, the surgeon should remember that the uterus is not the cause of uterovaginal prolapse. Uterine prolapse is the result but not the cause. Performing a hysterectomy will not solve the problem of prolapse. Indeed, it may not be absolutely necessary to remove the uterus in all cases. Removal of the uterus will facilitate repair of an enterocele [removing the uterus causes enterocele]†. Leaving the uterus in place can facilitate repair of a cystocele. Support for the vaginal walls, vaginal vault, and vaginal outlet is the most important part of the operation, not hysterectomy, although it is generally desirable to remove the uterus for other reasons.

The doctors continue with their "principles"—all procedures mentioned will be explained later in this chapter:

- "The surgeon should repair all relaxations, even though they are minor."
- "Whenever possible the surgeon should attempt to recreate normal anatomy."

---

† *Author's note*

- "The cul-de-sac should be closed and enteroceles repaired in all cases."

- "A posterior colpoperineorrhaphy [rectocele repair] should be performed in all cases."

- "The urethrovesical [bladder neck] angle should be supported separately to correct or prevent genuine stress urinary incontinence."

- "It is especially important to do a Burch suprapubic colpourethropexy [bladder neck suspension] when a sacral colpopexy [vaginal vault suspension] is performed."

- "It is also important to do an anterior colporrhaphy [cystocele repair] when the vaginal vault is suspended to the sacrospinous ligament."

- "The surgeon should make an independent decision about each part of the operation."

The "principles" conclude with a quote from Victor Bonney, a gynecologist practicing in the early part of the twentieth century, stressing that the surgeon should try:

In the words of Gilbert's immortal Lord High Executioner, "to make the punishment fit the crime'" by employing just those dissections, excisions, re-adjustments, and suturings that will, if possible, leave the parts concerned 'as good as new.'[3]

American pelvic surgery began in 1809 with a drastic and risky operation performed on Christmas Day in Danville, Kentucky. Ephraim McDonald (1771–1830) removed a twenty pound ovarian cyst from the swollen abdomen of a young woman whose relatives, it is told, were waiting outside ready to lynch the physician if his experiment failed. Miraculously, his knowledge and insight proved successful in removing the cyst without anesthesia or a sterile environment, and the woman quickly recovered to eventually outlive the surgeon. While this pioneering feat had all the elements of good medicine: caring, courage, competence, responsiveness, and good intent, a much darker story emerges next from the archives of surgical history.

James Marion Sims (1813–1883) often referred to as the "father of gynecology," lived in the South where he developed his surgical skills by operating on black slave women whom he kept in a barn behind his house. These experiments were performed over a four-year period without anesthesia and repeatedly on the same women. His own friends begged him to stop, and when his colleagues abandoned him, he trained other black slaves as assistants.

What Sims was working so hard to perfect was the repair of vesicovaginal fistula (VVF), a rare condition in which an opening occurs between the vagina and the bladder. As it so happens, Sims was a strong advocate of pessaries and, in fact, was in the pessary business himself. He fashioned pessaries from "block tin or gutta-percha softened with a little lead," and fit them individually to each of his patients. A connection between his lead pessaries and the high numbers of fistula he treated was almost certainly more than coincidental. An increased incidence of obstructed labor must also have been responsible for such high rates of vesicovaginal fistula, as is frequently witnessed in many African countries today. The reason for this is that girls are forced into marriage and sexual intercourse years before pelvic growth is complete, causing damage to pelvic organs as well as high-risk labor and delivery. Rickets, a disease caused by vitamin D deficiency, is the most common cause of inlet contraction, a condition where the bony birth passage is too small to accommodate the fetal head. Obstructed labor can result in maternal death, fetal death, and severe injury to pelvic structures.

Sims relocated to New York during the Civil War where he became chief of gynecology at The Woman's Hospital. He continued his surgical experiments on both rich and poor alike. One woman, Mary Smith, an Irish indigent, suffered thirty of his operations between 1856 and 1859. This was the same number the black slave Anarcha suffered at his hands ten years before.[4] Thus began a surgical furor that would continue to the present, for, "The repair of vesicovaginal fistulas and the removal of ovaries for a wide variety of indications were the beginning of the field of operative gynecology as it is known today."[5]

The last years of the nineteenth century and the first decades of the twentieth century continued the Great Experiment in gynecologic surgery. Uterine suspensions were very much in vogue during this period for all manner of pelvic complaints. Surgeons had absolute autonomy to perform any operation they could conceive of. The eminent gynecologist Howard Kelly (1858–1943), who founded the gynecology department at Johns Hopkins University (still a leading institution in experimental female pelvic surgery), described more than fifty uterine suspension operations; his colleague Hadden described one-hundred and twenty.[6] Dismal failure rates caused most surgeons to abandon suspension operations in favor of disposing of the uterus entirely with hysterectomy. The results of the drastic effects of hysterectomy on the pelvic interior led to the development of hundreds of variations of other operations for prolapse and incontinence that today make up 60 percent of the gynecological caseload.

Surgeries for Pelvic Organ Prolapse

Vaginal Hysterectomy

Although hysterectomy has been sharply criticized from both within and outside the gynecologic industry for close to a century, it remains the treatment of choice for uterine prolapse and many other benign pelvic conditions. Surgeons have become increasingly enthusiastic about vaginal hysterectomy (surgically removing the uterus through vaginal dissection instead of through abdominal dissection) in recent decades, convincing three generations of women that a "simple" vaginal operation will relieve them of a useless, painful, aggravating, and potentially dangerous organ.

Vaginal hysterectomy for pelvic organ prolapse is no longer recommended as a single operation due to the high incidence of post-hysterectomy vaginal vault prolapse. This situation results from the vagina having lost its supportive connections to the cervix and uterine ligaments, often turning completely inside out and hanging out of the vaginal opening. So in addition to vaginal hysterectomy, a surgeon may choose to perform one or several additional operations at the same time, including anterior colporrhaphy, posterior colporrhaphy, culdoplasty, and sacrocolpopexy or sacrospinous ligament fixation. If a woman is older and states she no longer desires sexual experience, or if the surgeon deems it necessary, her vagina may be completely removed (colpectomy) or her vaginal walls sutured shut (colpocleisis).

The hysterectomy begins with traction applied to the cervix, pulling it all the way down the vaginal canal. An incision is made through the vaginal layers surrounding the cervix and continues lengthwise on both sides toward the uterine fundus. The front vaginal wall and the bladder are retracted upward in order to further open the incision and to view the peritoneum (tissue that encases the abdominal cavity) from which the uterus is amputated. The back vaginal wall is then dissected from the cervix, uterus, and posterior peritoneum. The uterosacral and cardinal ligaments are clamped, cut, and sewn closed first on one side, then on the other. The uterus is pulled through the back peritoneal opening, severed from the uteroovarian and round ligaments, and the hysterectomy is complete at this point.

If the ovaries and fallopian tubes are to be removed as well, one tube and ovary is grasped with forceps, amputated from the clamped infundibulopelvic ligament, and pulled free from the pelvic cavity. The procedure is repeated on the other side. A large opening now exists between the top of the vagina and the interior of the abdomen. The surgeon closes the abdominal peritoneum first, which must be trimmed of excess tissue that once attached to the uterus. The shortened vaginal vault is then closed with sutures that pass through both the vaginal apex and the ligament stumps in hopes of creating adequate support for the vagina.

In spite of recent scientific evidence that the uterus secretes substances throughout our lifetime that control pain, stabilize mood, and mediate cardiovascular function,[7] hysterectomy remains gynecology's first course of treatment for many benign conditions. Describing the effects of hysterectomy on the pelvic interior, Nora Coffey, president of the HERS Foundation, tells us that the uterus is:

Attached to a major blood supply and a large bundle of nerves. When the ligaments that attach to the uterus are severed they are then hanging at one end and tied in bundles, no longer attached to anything at the other end. Those are the supporting ligaments for the entire pelvic structure. When those ligaments are severed, it permits the pelvis to broaden and widen. It is not an old wives tale that women become broader across the pelvis and backside after hysterectomy, it is a reality. One of the effects of severing the ligaments is that you lose the natural movement and sway of your hips, and develop a frozen pelvis. When the blood supply to the uterus is severed you lose much of the sensation and many women lose all sensation to the vagina, clitoris and nipples. Many women also have at the site at which the nerves were severed, chronic pain and inflammation of the nerve endings.[8]

The blood supply to the ovaries, uterus, and vagina comes directly off the great iliac arteries branching from the aorta of the heart. Although the ovaries and uterus have their own branches from these larger vessels, these merge into what surgeons call a "continuous arterial arcade" connecting this blood supply all along the sides of the ovaries, tubes, uterus, and vagina (Figure 4-1).[9]

Removing the uterus is cutting away the heart of this arterial and venous blood flow to the ovaries and vagina. Not only is their major blood supply disrupted, but also their nerve conduction and lymphatic drainage.

Of utmost importance structurally are the broad ligaments of the uterus, which wall off both the

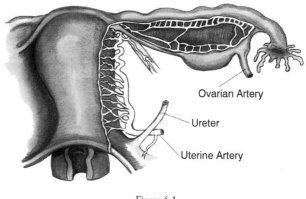

Figure 4-1
Blood Supply to the Uterus, Ovaries & Vagina

bladder and rectum, preventing these organs from severe and intractable prolapse (see Figure 13-5). The broad ligaments are destroyed during all forms of hysterectomy.

Anterior Colporrhaphy

The most common site of loss of pelvic organ support is the front wall of the vagina. Remember that the entire pelvic cavity is held together by a continuous system of connective tissue. When this tissue lengthens, widens, and thickens it is called ligament. When it is the strong, fibrous membrane surrounding pelvic organs it is referred to as endopelvic fascia. Even though doctors diagnose and treat specific pelvic floor "defects," it is easy to understand that pelvic relaxation does not occur in isolation; it must be considered within a broader context of female pelvic anatomy.

When normal pelvic anatomy changes, either as a result of pregnancy and childbirth or postural and lifestyle habits, the focus of intra-abdominal pressure shifts, weakening fascial support usually in one primary area and other secondary areas. The widely published pelvic surgeon Bobby L. Shull states "None of my patients have had isolated prolapse of the uterus or vaginal cuff without associated pelvic support defects involving the anterior or posterior segments of the vagina."[10]

When the pelvic support system begins to weaken, the urethra and bladder are often the first to pull back from their original positions and fall against the front vaginal wall. This causes a vaginal bulge that in some cases protrudes outside the introitus. As we saw in the last chapter, the angle at which the bladder descends determines the type of symptom that will result. If the bladder neck and lower urethra lose their normal axis, pressure closing of the urethra no longer takes place resulting in intermittent stress urinary incontinence. If the large base of the bladder falls into the vagina, there is often not a problem with incontinence, but rather with complete emptying of the bladder. Residual urine left in the bladder predisposes a woman to chronic bladder infection, or cystitis.

Anterior colporrhaphy, commonly referred to as "anterior repair," is one of the oldest and most venerated procedures in operative gynecology. Although surgeons are aware that "Patients with cystocele who have mild degrees of genuine stress urinary incontinence may be improved or even cured by pelvic floor musculature exercises,"[11] they are taught in the same breath that anterior colporrhaphy "is a useful operation for curing mild to moderate degrees of genuine stress urinary incontinence."[12] In cases of cystocele, the goal of the operation is to reduce the vaginal bulge and to correct any accompanying stress incontinence.

The technique consists of dissecting the front wall of the vagina open from the very top (apex) to within one centimeter of the external urethral meatus (where urine exits the body). The fascial attachments (which some sources say are not really discernible from vaginal tissue) behind the vaginal wall and just under the bladder and urethra are dissected to each side.[13] Beginning at the urethral meatus, the cut edges of fascia are plicated, or re-gathered together, and stitched at the midline. The stitches pull the tissue edges together tightly and, as they do so, raise the urethra. The plication is continued to the bladder neck where the sutures are anchored on either side into ligaments behind the pubic bone. A strip of vagina is removed from either side of the incision, the edges brought back together tighter than they were before, and sewn closed. A urinary catheter is inserted to monitor bladder drainage for several days post-op.

Anterior colporrhaphy is still widely practiced just as Howard Kelly described it in 1914 although it has one of the poorest success rates of all pelvic reconstructive surgeries. One prospective study found the surgery to have alleviated symptoms of urinary stress incontinence in 63 percent of women at one year post-op, and 37 percent of those same women five years after the procedure.[14] Another study found the cure rate for anterior colporrhaphy to be 45 percent at one to two years, and 31 percent at five years.[15] Yet another study using various novel techniques and state of the art technology still only yielded success rates between 42 percent and 57 percent. When anterior colporrhaphy is performed for an asymptomatic large cystocele, up to 80 percent of patients return with surgically induced incontinence.[16]

Complications include urethral obstruction due to bands of tightened vaginal scar tissue compressing the bladder. This leads to symptoms of urinary urgency, bladder spasms, a slow urinary stream, straining to void, and a feeling of incomplete emptying.[17] Various studies have reported recurrence rates of cystocele after anterior colporrhaphy to be between three percent and thirty-three percent.[18] Women report difficulties with a narrowed vagina, pain with intercourse, and loss of vaginal and clitoral sensation.

Although every imaginable surgical strategy has been employed to address prolapse of the front vaginal wall, surgical management of cystocele remains problematic. "Cystoceles, although a common clinical diagnosis, present a significant challenge for those treating pelvic floor disorders. They may be considered the nemesis of the pelvic surgeon."[19] Many surgeons are using polypropylene mesh overlays between the vaginal wall and bladder in an attempt to fortify the repair. These prosthetics often reduce cystocele, but yield erosion rates between thirteen percent to twenty-five percent.[20]

For decades, doctors have recognized the dismal effects of vaginal dissection on pelvic organ support. Technological developments to support this reality can now measure and provide evidence of the damage. Sensitive testing, including *perineal nerve terminal motor latency studies, single fiber electromyography, and muscle histochemistry,* confirm that gross disruption of vaginal integrity has significant, long-term, and detrimental effects on the nerve supply to both large and small muscles of the perineum.[21-23] This nerve damage is understood to be a major cause of loss of pelvic organ support, including urinary and fecal incontinence.[24-28] Studies have demonstrated that damage to the pudendal nerve is present in women with pelvic organ descent and stress incontinence.[29] Vaginal dissection does not improve the preconditions of stress incontinence and pelvic relaxation, but rather causes worsening of pre-existing pudendal nerve damage (the nerve supply to the urethra), continuing the cycle of dysfunction and surgery.[30-32] Despite debilitating complications and high recurrence rates, hundreds of thousands of these operations are performed annually in the United States because there remain virtually no objective, long-term studies of their anatomical and functional results.

Posterior Colporrhaphy

Rectocele is a common condition amongst Western women. Although symptoms of rectocele occur in young women who have never been pregnant, this disorder is more likely to manifest in the weeks and months following vaginal delivery.

Nearly two-thirds of all women who give birth in American hospitals choose to be anesthetized from the waist down (Figure 4-2). This anesthesia is known to slow the labor process, particularly in the second

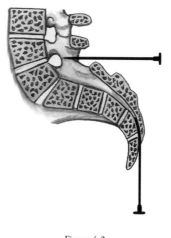

Figure 4-2
Spinal Anesthesia

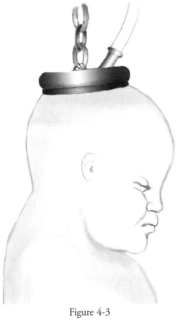

Figure 4-3
Vacuum Extraction

stage when the baby's head is pressing against the pelvic diaphram.[33-37] When the woman is lying on her back (lithotomy position), which is the routine position for hospital delivery, the pressure is against the rectovaginal septum. Prolonged second stage of labor is cited as a common contributor to the development of pelvic organ prolapse, as are vacuum extractions (Figure 4-3) and forceps deliveries (Figure 4-4).[38-40]

More and more women and their doctors are choosing to schedule when delivery will take place by inducing labor with oxytocic hormones. A study by the National Institutes of Health found the rate of labor induction more than doubled from 1990 to 1998, more than 50 percent of which were elective.[41] Inducing labor with synthetic hormones begins a cascade of obstetric intervention, including continuous fetal heart monitoring, early epidural anesthesia due to heightened discomfort from speeded-up contractions, episiotomy, instrumental delivery, and increased risk of cesarean section.

Episiotomy is the most common surgery performed on the perineum. It is also the only surgery performed without consent of the patient. In at least 40 percent of women giving birth in American hospitals[42] (down from over 60 percent a decade ago), a carefully timed incision is made into the perineal body for the alleged purpose of either aiding the actual delivery process or preventing perineal tears. If the incision is made too early, before the fetal head is pressing on the perineum, there is severe bleeding as blood vessels run parallel with nerve vessels throughout this area.

The incision is made in one of two ways, either midline (Figure 4-5) from the vagina to just before the anus, or mediolateral (Figure 4-6), an angled cut from the vagina toward the side of the anus. All too frequently during birth, midline episiotomies extend or keep tearing to what is called a third degree injury (into the anus) or a fourth degree injury (into the rectum) (Figure 4-7). These are extremely serious wounds

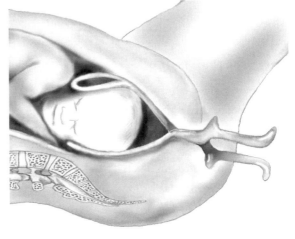

Figure 4-4
Forceps Delivery

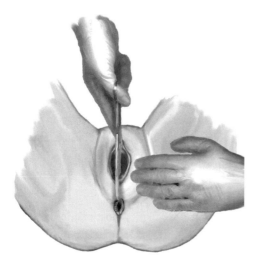

Figure 4-5
Midline Episiotomy

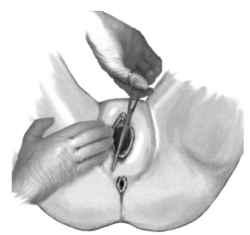

Figure 4-6
Medialateral Episiotomy

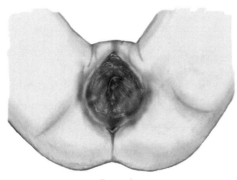

Figure 4-7
4th Degree Episiotomy Wound

that require months of care, powerful antibiotic therapy, and sometimes two and three attempts at surgical closure. Midline episiotomy predisposes women to rectal injury. Mediolateral episiotomy does not protect against rectal injury[43] and is bloodier, more painful, slower to heal, very disfiguring, and just as damaging to the nerve supply of the perineum.[44] Certain races of women, most notably Asian women, are known to have a very short perineum, or little space between the introitus and anal sphincter. Routine episiotomy performed on these women significantly heightens their risk of sustaining severe injury to the anus and bowel. Serious tearing of the perineum during natural childbirth is rare, and several recent studies have revealed that episiotomy not only carries significant risk of damage to the rectum and anal sphincter, but also is associated with a permanently disfigured perineum, painful intercourse, rectovaginal fistula, infection, pelvic organ prolapse, and death.[45-53]

Since 1953 obstetricians and gynecologists have known of the relationship between episiotomy and stress urinary incontinence:

Any perineal laceration which permits the labia minora to retract laterally and expose a gaping vagina harbors the divided and retracted origin of the bulbocavernousus muscle. Such a lesion lowers the efficiency of the voluntary urethral sphincter and should be considered as an etiologic basis for stress urinary incontinence in the female.[54]

A recent study found a significant increase in perineal body measurement from the first to the third trimester, a clear indication of natural protection against anal sphincter injury and perineal body destruction.[55] The long-term effects of episiotomy are once again being considered by scientific medicine:

> *Destruction of the perineal body and alteration of the [pelvic floor] muscles comprise the first pathophysiological events in the natural history of genital prolapse. The buffer of the core of the perineal body disappears. Once the puborectalis muscle has been thinned or weakened, the urogenital hiatus becomes widely open. The ventral vaginal wall sticks out. It pulls the uterine cervix downward, reduces the physiological anteversion of the uterine body and facilitates eversion.*[56]

According to a report in the *Journal of Reproductive Medicine*, most residents in obstetrics and gynecology receive little or no formal instruction in how to repair an episiotomy, and only about 28 percent of residents are supervised by an attending physician when repairing "relatively complicated" episiotomies. The report states, "So we have doctors with no supervision who also are seeing less and therefore doing less, which compounds the potential problem for women if the doctors don't have good, basic anatomy training."[57] Costa Rican midwife Doña Miriam Elizondo, age eighty, estimates she has attended more than two thousand natural births, and has never had a fatal outcome. Pondering why in the world obstetricians perform routine episiotomies, she reflects, "The part stretches beautifully, just like elastic!"[58]

Although modern childbirth accounts for most rectoceles, others result from lifestyle habits such as diet and straining against the hard rim of the toilet seat. The medical literature cites again and again as contributing factors, constipation and straining with bowel movements, yet rarely are these issues properly addressed as causes of the problem.

Posterior colporrhaphy, referred to as "posterior repair," is surgical correction of a rectocele. It begins with a midline incision at the back vaginal wall from the perineum to the top of the vagina and often laterally from one side of the vagina to the other. The wall is dissected from its fascial attachments and sutured to deeper endopelvic fascia and sometimes to surrounding musculature. If there is not enough fascia to plicate, which is frequently the case, a mass of levator muscle is gathered and stitched together down the midline of the vagina and perineum to form a firm barricade between vagina and rectum. The vaginal wall is trimmed, pulled together more tightly, and sewn closed, while the posterior aspect of the vaginal opening and bulbocavernosos muscles are stitched transversely by perineorrhaphy in an attempt to create a new perineal body.

Posterior colporrhaphy is another very old operation dating from the nineteenth century and does not address the cause or prevention of rectocele. The goal of the operation is to eliminate the symptom, or bulge, into the back wall of the vagina. It is also one of the least successful and most damaging of all operations for pelvic relaxation, leading one surgeon to comment, "A repair that focuses on eliminating the vaginal bulge without normalizing rectal defects or addressing associated symptoms seems to be treating the gynecologists observations, rather than the patient's concerns."[59] It was demonstrated in 1932, and subsequently reported in a famous scientific paper, that no muscle fibers of the levator ani ever cross the midline.[60] Rather, they part like hair down the middle of a scalp. Therefore, it is quite unnatural to have a midline scar in this area. Many sutures have to be placed into the levator muscles that have been gathered and folded together. This causes a severe inflammatory response leading to gross scar formation.[61] The resulting thick, unyielding band of scar tissue between vagina and rectum often makes sexual intercourse permanently painful.[62,63] This has been known for many decades as have the worsening of other symptoms after surgery such as defecatory function, constipation, incomplete emptying of the rectum, and fecal incontinence.[64,65] Extreme nerve damage, combined with reconfiguring of the levator muscles into a bulky mass, causes the perineum to descend even further, creating an ever more vicious cycle of nerve damage and loss of pelvic organ support.

Some surgeons have advocated locating and repairing only isolated, site-specific tears in the rectovaginal fascia in place of full midline plication. However, little difference in outcome has been noted between the two techniques.

> *Throughout the years, the diagnosis and management of rectocele has been an uncomfortable arena for the pelvic surgeon. The results have been disappointing and in many places rectocele repair has given rise to more dissatisfaction than satisfaction, and the procedure has been abandoned.*[66]

As with anterior repair, in recent years synthetic mesh has been utilized to augment tissue repair in the back vaginal wall. Studies have since demonstrated that the use of mesh in the vagina has not improved the outcome of rectocele repair and is associated with significant complications.

Sacrospinous Ligament Fixation

In some cases of vaginal hysterectomy, the ligament stumps are determined to be too weak to adequately support the vagina. A testament to this fact can be found in the high percentage of post-hysterectomy prolapse of the vaginal vault. Without the uterus and especially the broad ligaments to hold it in place, the vagina may turn completely inside out and hang out of the body. The incidence of vaginal vault prolapse after abdominal or vaginal hysterectomy is said to range from 0.2 percent to 45 percent.[67,68]

Correction of post-hysterectomy vaginal vault prolapse is a late-stage attempt to treat the difficult problem of surgically induced pelvic system collapse. At least forty-three different operations are described in the medical literature that use vaginal, abdominal, and laparoscopic approaches to the problem.[69] A popular treatment of choice in vaginal vault prolapse is sacrospinous ligament fixation, or more appropriately transvaginal sacrospinous colpopexy.

This surgery begins with an incision through the perineum and back vaginal wall to enter the space between vagina and rectum. The rectum is retracted to one side to allow for dissection deep into the pelvis to what is called the pararectal space. At the sides of this space deep behind the rectum lie the sacrospinous ligaments and coccygeal muscles, which connect the sacrum (bottom of the spinal column) to the rest of the pelvic musculature. More retraction and tunneling with the scalpel exposes the sacrospinous ligaments.

The surgeon must be very careful to avoid endangering the sciatic and pudendal nerves and vessels, which also traverse this area. The ligament is grasped with a long clamp and threaded with sutures that are then sewn through one side of the vaginal vault. The procedure may or may not be repeated on the other side, depending upon whether the vaginal stump is long enough to reach to both sacrospinous ligaments. Closure of the back of the vagina is begun from the top to the middle, where the sacrospinous colpopexy stitches are then securely tied, firmly attaching the vagina to the sacrospinous ligament. The vagina and perineum are then stitched closed.

Transvaginal fixation of the vault to the sacrospinous ligament is fraught with difficulties and exposes women to potential damage to the pudendal vessels, sciatic nerve damage, and injury to the urinary tract and rectum. In addition, the vagina is no longer compliant and mobile, but shortened and held taut in an exaggerated angle toward the sacrum, impairing sexual function. This constant pulling of the vagina toward the back predisposes women to problems in the front wall of the vagina.[70-76] Various studies have reported up to a 92 percent occurrence of cystocele after sacrospinous ligament fixation, yet not a single study exists in all of medical literature examining the long-term effects of having the muscular vagina permanently tethered to one side of the spine.[77]

Abdominal Sacrocolpopexy

An abdominal approach to this same problem is commonly attempted in a procedure called abdominal sacrocolpopexy. Here, after dissection through the abdominal cavity, the vaginal vault is suspended from the front surface of the sacrum using a "natural" (from pigs, cadavers or the patient's own tissue) or synthetic mesh material between the apex of the vagina and the anterior ligament of the sacrum. Many complications are associated with this surgery, including stress urinary incontinence with or without a prophylactic continence procedure, recurrent cystocele, mesh erosion into the vagina, infection, bowel dysfunction, severe hemorrhage, sacral osteomyelitis (bone infection), and death.[78-82] There are no established criteria for choosing the abdominal over vaginal route, nor is there any reliable data comparing the outcomes of abdominal sacrocolpopexy and sacrospinous vault suspension.[83] The durability of the operation appears to decrease over time, which may have to do with the fact that the anterior ligament undergoes age-related changes: "Its energy-absorbing and elastic properties decrease with age, as does the strength of the bone into which it is attached. As the mineral content of the surrounding bone decreases with age, the strength of the ligament also decreases."[84] The sacrum must be dissected from the connective tissues that envelop it, and the sacral artery identified and carefully avoided. One surgeon describes the consequences of accidentally cutting into the sacral artery:

> The potential for significant hemorrhage that is almost impossible to stop exists with this approach. If major bleeding occurs, hemostasis by suturing is almost impossible. Usually pressure for 10 to 15 minutes stops the bleeding. If this does not work, a sterile thumbtack with bone wax nailed into the sacrum works.[85]

No medical studies exist that examine the long-term outcome of having the sacral spine permanently tethered to the vaginal stump.

Surgeries for Uterine Prolapse

Successfully replacing a prolapsed uterus in a correct anatomic position has always been and remains an unsolved piece of the pelvic surgery puzzle.[86] For more than a century, countless surgical strategies have been tried: all have failed. Most have been abandoned in favor of total hysterectomy. One of the greatest wonders of the female pelvic support system is that this keystone, the uterus, which only plays a passive role in its own descent, actually acts as a deterrent to all other forms of pelvic organ prolapse.[87]

Perhaps there is a relationship between this unsolvable problem and the reason why for decades we've been told uterine descent is a disease of older women, that it is a serious condition, and one that is only corrected by hysterectomy. Current studies are beginning to reveal what gynecologists have always known, that pelvic organ prolapse is a disorder of young, healthy women as well as "little old ladies."[88]

Better informed of the serious consequences of hysterectomy, women suffering with uterine prolapse are demanding surgeries that correct prolapse while preserving the uterus. Gynecologists and urogynecologists have taken note of recent trends and are again offering uterine suspensions as viable solutions to prolapse. Many surgical techniques are available, some new, but most are renditions of the same operations abandoned long ago due to high failure rates and morbid complications.

Uterosacral Ligament Suspension

Initial observations of the uterosacral ligaments during the early years of the twentieth century concluded these were not important support structures of the uterus.[89] Later researchers argued that while the ligaments have some surgical usefulness, they should not be "credited with undue supportive value." The uterosacral ligaments are described as "condensations of pelvic cellular tissue around vessels and nerves" concluding that it is unlikely "under physiologic conditions the ligaments that primarily convey the pelvic parasympathetic nerve fibers from the sacral plexus to the lateral aspects of the uterus have significant supportive function."[90,91] Nevertheless, laparoscopic plication of the uterosacral ligaments has become the most popular uterine suspension operation performed in modern times.

This procedure places a series of permanent sutures bilaterally through the ligament complex and into the fascia covering the posterior side of the cervix. The uterosacral ligaments are thus said to be "shortened" and "strengthened," as the uterus is raised to a more anatomically correct level. No reliable studies exist on the outcomes of uterosacral ligament suspension. However, recent data has shed new light on what pelvic surgeons have long suspected, that plication of these ligaments can cause injury to the S1-S4 trunks of the sacral nerve plexus:

> *Our findings suggest that suture injury is anatomically plausible. We do not know how often this complication occurs but we suspect that it may be underdiagnosesd. Suture injury to the sacral plexes trunks S1-S4 can result in damage to nerve fibers in (1) the nerve to the quadratus femoris and the gemellus inferior; (2) the nerve to the obturator internus and gemellus superior; (3) the nerve to the piriformis; (4) the nerves to the superior and inferior gluteus; (5) the posterior femoral cutaneous nerve; (6) the pudendal nerve; and (7) the sciatic truck and its branches to the thigh, leg, and foot. Clinically, this would present as sensory loss involving the S1-S4 cutaneous dermatomes of the perineum and the lower extremity. Possible areas of motor weakness would occur with hip extension and abduction, knee flexion, and plantar flexion.*[92]

Ventrosuspension of the Uterus

Several variations on this operation strive to tighten the round ligaments and hold the uterus in its normal, forward-facing position. The procedure can now be performed laparoscopically, but typically it is done using a low abdominal incision. The rectus muscle of the abdomen is first dissected from its fascial sheath. A long tweezer-like instrument is punctured through the abdominal wall and the round ligament grasped, pulled through, and secured to the inside of the rectus fascia with permanent sutures. This shortens the round ligaments, tilting the uterus forward.

Surgical procedures that rely on support from the round ligaments have dismally high failure rates. The round ligaments are composed primarily of smooth muscle cells, which make them inherently weak.[93] Pain with exercise is a known complication, but ventrosuspension creates a far more ominous possibility for future problems.

Fixing the round ligament to the inside of the abdominal wall creates a tunnel between the layers of muscle and fascia. This tunnel widens with time resulting in a hole through which a section of small bowel can herniate, obstruct, and eventually strangulate. New Zealand shares with us the awesome fact that major gynecologic surgery is responsible for 12 percent of their hospital admissions with subacute bowel obstruction and up to 60 percent of cases of bowel obstruction requiring emergency surgery. Twenty percent of these events occur up to 10 years after the original surgery.[94]

Hysterocolposacropexy

This version of abdominal colposacropexy preserves the uterus by joining the connective tissue surrounding it with the sacrum by way of a synthetic mesh graft. It carries the same surgical risks as colposacropexy with the added risk, in the event of future hysterectomy, of great difficulty dissecting the deeply embedded mesh from the sacrum. [95] Yet, hysterocolposacropexy is becoming the "gold standard" of uterine suspension surgeries.

It is completely legal for doctors to sell surgical procedures to women as "cures" for prolapse even though the operations are also associated with gross complications. One of the few uterine suspension studies, in which twenty-nine women ages twenty-nine to forty-three years were observed between 1987 and 1999, concluded that "Hysterocolposacropexy seems to be the operation of choice for the correction of uterovaginal prolapse in women of childbearing age. This procedure has a high cure rate without a time dependent decrease inefficiency,"[96] even though one woman experienced hemorrhage of the presacral veins and one a hematoma during surgery; two developed new-onset pain with intercourse; one developed mesh erosion; one an intestinal blockage; one an incision-related abdominal hernia; one a recurrent urinary tract infection; and one chronic sciatic nerve pain.

Surgeries for Urinary Incontinence

Leaking small amounts of urine during increases in intra-abdominal pressure is one of the most common complaints women bring to the gynecologist. stress urinary incontinence can be either transitory, meaning it can disappear on its own, or it can worsen over time.[97] The determining factor in whether incontinence will improve or worsen is the total health of the pelvic organ support system.

Years of allowing the spine and pelvis to assume unhealthy postures cause the levator plate at the back of the pelvis to weaken and sag creating a steeper than normal angle of the genital hiatus (Figure 4-8). It is through this hiatus that the pelvic organs fall. Often it is the urethra and neck of the bladder that first begin to be pulled down through the hiatus. Although there are many causes of urinary incontinence, from instability of the bladder muscle to neurological damage, the vast majority of urogynecologic surgeries performed are to relieve symptoms of stress urinary

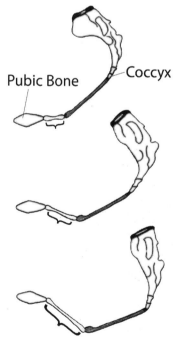

Figure 4-8
Progressive Widening of the Genital Hiatus

incontinence. Over one hundred different surgical procedures have been used to treat the symptoms of stress incontinence. No ideal method has been found and all procedures are said to have a failure rate of between 15 percent and 50 percent.[98] Female urinary incontinence affects up to 38 percent of women, and "Despite the extent of this problem, there have been few advances in the treatment of this disorder."[99]

Retropubic Bladder Neck Suspension

An abdominal approach to stabilize the urethra and bladder neck, formally called retropubic urethropexy, was first described by Marshall, Marchetti, and Krantz in 1949. This and many variations of the original operation are performed in an attempt to stabilize the urethra by attaching the endopelvic fascia surrounding the urethra to various fixed points behind the pubic bone. The classic Marshall, Marchetti, and Krantz (MMK) procedure places a series of sutures along the urethra and bladder neck, then drives the needle directly into the pubic bone. The original technique has since been modified (although it is still performed) because sutures placed in the pubic bone put women at risk for developing osteitis pubis, an extremely painful, debilitating inflammatory disease.

The operation begins by preparing both the vagina and the abdomen for surgery. A catheter is placed in the bladder and a horizontal incision is made close to the pubic bone. The incision goes down through the fascia to the rectus muscles of the abdomen, which are dissected from their insertion points onto the pubic bone. The surgeon then enters an area behind the pubic bone called the space of Retzius. When thoroughly dissected, this space reveals the back of the pubis and associated ligaments, the endopelvic fascia, the urethra and bladder, and the vaginal wall.

With one hand in the vagina to push up and make more visible the endopelvic fascia, the surgeon uses his other hand to hook two to four sutures into this fascia. The sutures are then fixed to the chosen anchor point and tied down. The rectus muscle is sewn closed; additional stitches close the rectus fascia. Subcutaneous stitches are made through the fat layers, and the skin is sewn closed and covered with steri-strips.

Retropubic bladder neck suspension is considered by many doctors to be the most successful method for surgically treating urinary stress incontinence. This is because the bladder neck is permanently elevated to a level that makes any leaking of urine virtually impossible. That gynecologists and urogynecologists can possibly claim this surgery a success (and indiscriminately sell it to their patients) is astonishing given the devastating array of other maladies the surgery creates. Surgeons have been aware for many decades of the complications associated with bladder neck suspensions, "Women who undergo retropubic urethropexy for urinary incontinence have an approximately 80 percent five-year cure rate for genuine stress incontinence but have only a 50 percent overall cure rate free of newly acquired voiding disabilities or pelvic organ prolapse."[100] Many studies have revealed voiding difficulties, bladder muscle instability, kinking of the urethra, recurrent bladder infections, pain with intercourse, enterocele, rectocele, and uterovaginal prolapse as significant post-surgical occurrences.[101-105]

Because of the unnaturally high position of the urethra and bladder neck, a woman who has had this surgery is cured of incontinence, but now has to strain each time she urinates. This creates undue pressure throughout the urinary tract, leading to kinking of the urethra (causing dribbling after urination), a hypersensitive bladder muscle (feeling like one has to urinate when the bladder is only slightly full), and eventually to an abnormal shape of the bladder itself.[106] The inability to push all urine out of the bladder can lead to recurrent bouts of cystitis.

In 1961 John Burch reported that Cooper's ligament, rather than the pubic bone, was a more acceptable place to connect the endopelvic fascia surrounding the urethra and bladder neck, this surgery being generally referred to as the Burch procedure ever since. Burch himself reported that the front wall of the vagina was pulled permanently forward with this surgery, predisposing women to enterocele, rectocele, and uterine prolapse.[107] A recent study found that the routinely performed combination of Burch urethropexy and posterior colporrhaphy was especially likely to result in painful sexual intercourse.[108]

Symptomatic enteroceles are rare in women who have not had pelvic surgery. It is when the uterus is removed or the vagina pulled forward that the cul-de-sac of Douglas becomes wider, allowing the bowel to fall down against the back wall of the vagina. Culdoplasty is often performed in conjunction with hysterectomy and bladder neck suspension surgeries. In this procedure the pouch of peritoneum (cul-de-sac) is stitched closed, thus eliminating this natural curve along the intestinal pathway. The incidence of uterovaginal prolapse after bladder suspension surgery has been variously reported to be between 7.6 percent and 66 percent.[109] A similar range of post-operative rectoceles and enteroceles has also been described.[110]

A group of Italian gynecologists recently submitted a paper to the *British Journal of Obstetrics and Gynaecology* that sums up the unfortunate situation of trying to correct pelvic floor weakness with surgery:

> *In light of our current data and of those reported elsewhere, we believe that the Burch colposuspension should no longer be performed in women with advanced anterior wall prolapse because the operation has an unacceptable high rate of prolapse recurrence. Concomitant abdominal hysterectomy, culdoplasty, and vaginal posterior repair seem to be of little value. On the other hand, continued use of the anterior colporrhaphy in women with stress incontinence cannot be justified as its functional results are expected to be very poor.[111]*

In 1934 the highly respected English physician Victor Bonney published an article in *The Journal of Obstetrics and Gynaecology of the British Empire* entitled, "The Principles That Should Underlie All Operations For Prolapse."[112] He correctly described not only normal anatomy of the female pelvic organ support system, but all compensatory abnormalities that occur with surgical procedures for prolapse and incontinence. These principles are repeatedly outlined in gynecology textbooks and throughout the medical literature. No board certified gynecologist or urogynecologist is unfamiliar with them. Implicit in Bonney's principles is the glaring truth that any organ within the female pelvis that is removed or repositioned in any way begins a cascade of dysfunction for which there is no favorable solution. Our most published pelvic surgeons continue to lament this reality: "If his [Bonney's] theory is accurate, we have predisposed all our patients to anterior defects in much the same way a high retropubic urethropexy predisposes a woman to defects in the posterior cul-de-sac."[113] Still, practitioners continue to ignore this reality, and women continue to suffer the consequences.

Alloplastic Slings

Like most other pelvic reconstructive surgeries, suburethral sling operations are very old, the first one developed in 1907. And, like most other pelvic surgeries, there have existed a myriad of variations all using the same concept of a constructed sling to support the urethra.

Until the last years of the twentieth century, correction of female stress urinary incontinence entailed support of the bladder neck. From 1989 to 1993 two researchers, Peter Petros from Australia and Ulf Ulmsten from Sweden, collaborated on a new vaginal procedure that places a strip of polypropylene mesh under the mid-portion of the urethra. In 1995 an international patent was filed on the surgical packet containing a curved needle, or trocar, used in the procedure, a strip of polypropylene mesh, and an antiseptic Betadine swipe. A market launch of tension-free vaginal tape (TVT) took place the following year at a price of US $500 for each packet.

By 2002 the manufacturer of tension-free vaginal tape, Gynecare (a division of Ethicon Inc. and Johnson & Johnson of Sommerville, NJ), had sold more than 350,000 units for use internationally and more than 110,000 units in the United States. Today more than 1,000,000 of these slings have been implanted in women.[114]

During the outpatient procedure, two small incisions are made in the abdomen just above the pubic bone. Next, a 1 centimeter midline incision is made in the front wall of the vagina starting 1.5 centimeter from the urethral opening and continuing upwards toward the bladder. Blunt scissors are used to create two small tunnels from the vaginal opening toward the abdominal incisions. Using a rigid catheter as a guide, the curved trocar tethered to the strip of polypropylene mesh is inserted into the vaginal opening, threaded up in between the bladder and pubic bone, and then pulled out the abdominal incisions. The same technique is carried out on the opposite side so that the mesh is brought up under the urethra in a U-shaped sling. When the mesh is determined to be positioned properly under the urethra, it is removed from the trocar. It is not sutured at either end, hence the term "tension-free." Scarring and fibrosis anchor the mesh into place. The correct route of insertion is just to the side of the center of the back of the pubic bone. Going too far later-ally risks "catastrophic" vascular injury to the femoral artery and epigastric vessels. Tak-ing the needle too far up risks puncturing the colon or small bowel. Too far central risks bladder and urethral injury.

Since their inception, there has been much speculation as to how mid-urethral slings actually work, but it is generally agreed that it is by way of an obstructive mechanism. Continence is achieved by the urethra being compressed against and kinked around the tape. Tension-free vaginal tapes have demonstrated superior success rates for curing stress urinary incontinence and are replacing retropubic urethropexies and bladder neck slings as the standard treatment for these disorders. Marketed to doctors and patients alike as a minimally invasive, simple procedure, more than twenty-five different tapes and trocars and many modifications have been promoted since the original tension-free vaginal tape. Yet, "Clear evidence that suburethral slings may be better or worse than other surgical or conservative management is lacking."[115]

Although tens of thousands of tension-free slings are being implanted in women ev-ery year, systematic reviews or follow-ups for complications are rare.

> *Apparently, there are no accepted definitions of what "complication" means…more important seems to be the lack of follow-up, thus loss of information on mid- and long-term complications for the surgeon in many national health care systems. This is of importance concerning UTI* [uterine tract infection], *prolapse and invasion of slings into the lower urinary tract that apparently increase with time.*[116]

Today, many surgeons will offer them to young, sexually active women as a first course of treatment for stress urinary incontinence.

The most common complication following tension-free vaginal tape procedures is bladder perforation, with an incidence as high as 20 percent. This is followed by bladder outlet obstruction (which requires cutting of the tape), hematoma, tape erosion into the urethra or bladder, tape extrusion into the vagina, and vascular or bowel injury. "These complications can be very serious as deaths have been reported after the tension-free vagi-nal tape procedure."[117]

In an attempt to avoid tunneling through the retropubic space where risk of blad-der, bowel, and major vascular injuries are theoretically higher, a trans-obturator (TOT) approach to the placement of tension-free slings was introduced in 2001. Like the ten-sion-free vaginal tape, this method begins with a small incision underneath the urethra followed by dissecting the vagina off its underlying fascial layer. Another incision is made in the groin over the obturator foramen of the pelvis and a curved needle threaded with polypropylene tape is passed between the two openings. The tape is brought up under-neath the urethra and cut off at the groin incisions.

Hailed as the least invasive approach to stress urinary incontinence, by 2004 26.9 per-cent of midurethral synthetic slings placed in European hospitals were the trans-obturator tape. The technique became widely and quickly accepted because of its high rate of success at resolving symptoms of stress urinary incontinence and the general belief that there are fewer intraoperative complications associated with the procedure. However, bladder perforation[118] and vesicovaginal fistula[119] have been noted. Far more disturbing are the twenty-one case reports of life-threatening postoperative soft tissue infection of the thigh and groin.[120] Anatomical studies have demonstrated that trans-obturator tape connects the vagina directly to the upper thigh through the obturator foramen.

Posterior intravaginal slingplasty is a new procedure for vaginal vault prolapse that begins on the exterior surfaces of the buttocks. A trocar threaded with a strip of polypropylene mesh is forged along either side of the anus and rectum, advanced deeply into the interior of the pelvis, and onto the vaginal vault. Serious complications associated with having the interior of the pelvis permanently tethered below the spine are being reported.

It used to be that sling operations were the end stage in a lengthy female pelvic surgery drama. By the time a sling operation was required for intractable urinary incontinence, a woman had endured hysterectomy, her ovaries removed (castration), at least one incontinence operation, and perhaps surgery for vaginal vault prolapse. The natural dynamics of her pelvis were completely and permanently destroyed, and this procedure was often the final surgical solution. She was cured of pelvic organ prolapse and urinary incontinence, yet had lost her ability to squat, sit cross-legged, spread her legs, or urinate and defecate without difficulty. She no longer desired sexual experience, was unable to have pain-free intercourse, and no longer felt sexual pleasure or achieved orgasm.

The outcomes of widely practiced surgeries that cause this level of human pain and suffering should at least be held up to the same degree of critical analysis as other areas of society such as law and science. They have not been.[121] Criminally few scientific studies have measured the effectiveness of surgical treatments for the very common conditions of female pelvic organ prolapse and incontinence. Surgeons Linda Brubaker and Theodore Saclarides speak to the dismal quality of "scientific studies" that currently fill the medical literature: "Failure to report sub-optimal surgical outcomes must stop; clinical outcomes, for better or worse, must be reported honestly."[122]

Doctors frequently report extremely high surgical success rates based on their own small clinical populations, but virtually no large, objective, prospective studies have been done in this area.[123,124] Available studies comparing the outcome of pelvic reconstructive surgeries are mainly descriptive and retrospective.[125] "Randomized prospective studies are badly needed to evaluate not only new procedures, but many of those now commonly performed for which no conclusive evidence exists that the outcomes are better than with more conservative measures. Patterns of treatment are so ingrained, however, that specialty groups seem unwilling to participate in clinical trials."[126] True risk factors and long-term outcomes of these operations remain unknown, doctors continue to dissect the female pelvis, and women are still led to believe they will be helped instead of harmed.

∽

More Problems With Surgery

There is an ecology of bad ideas, just as there is an ecology of weeds, and it is character-istic of the system that basic error propagates itself. It branches out like a rooted parasite through the tissues of life, and everything gets into a rather peculiar mess.

GREGORY BATESON
Steps Toward an Ecology of Mind[1]

THE HARM TO WOMEN TAKING PLACE here and abroad as the practice of surgery for loss of pelvic organ support becomes institutionalized around the world is incalculable. Urogynecologists are the younger set of gynecologists whose practice is focused in large part on pelvic floor "dysfunction." Pelvic reconstructive surgery is an elite specialty unlike other surgical specialties. For it has developed from an iatrogenic (medically induced) foundation. The field of gynecology/urogynecology has built not only a practice but also a theoretical framework around pelvic reconstructive surgery based on failure to re-establish natural anatomy after surgical removal and/or repositioning of female pelvic organs.

Their "principles" allow them to work backward from a surgical ideal that has the uterus removed, the bladder sutured to the abdominal wall,† and the vagina shortened, narrowed, immobilized, and pulled in two directions at once. The "logic" with which surgeons approach the whole issue of loss of pelvic organ support is not logical at all. It is a highly lucrative circular chase of a normal process affecting, according to one study, 44 percent of women ages twenty to fifty-nine who have given birth and 30.8 percent of all women ages twenty to fifty-nine years old[2] by a damaging, disfiguring, unsuccessful, and scientifically unsound precept. Let us identify a starting point in the circle chase and see where the doctors' reckoning takes us. The following quotations are all from the most revered gynecology journals and texts:

- "Many women after vaginal delivery have some degree of 'prolapse' (i.e. physical examination changes consistent with less than perfect vaginal support). Although this might be considered 'normal' for parous women [women who have given birth], we recommend that until data are available on which to base such

---

† *Cooper's ligament is just below the abdominal wall – still a ventrosuspension. In my own case it was the muscle of my abdominal wall that the fascia around my bladder was sutured to.*

a distinction, only the complete absence of prolapse should be considered 'normal'."[3]

- "The etiology [cause] of pelvic floor dysfunction remains poorly understood."[4]

- "Pudendal nerve damage and soft tissue trauma during the process of vaginal delivery has been demonstrated to be of etiologic importance in the development of urinary and fecal incontinence."[5]

- "Further epidemiologic studies are needed to determine the risk factors for pelvic organ prolapse."[6]

- "Such studies are difficult to conduct because of the long time intervals between the occurrence of presumed risk factors (such as vaginal delivery and hysterectomy) and the clinical presentation of pelvic floor dysfunction."[7]

- "Given the poor understanding of symptoms related to pelvic floor dysfunction, it frequently is difficult to counsel patients regarding which of their symptoms will improve with treatment."[8]

- "The lifetime risk of undergoing a single operation for pelvic organ prolapse and urinary incontinence is 11.1 percent."[9]

- "Subjects who have undergone surgery to correct pelvic organ prolapse should be viewed as already having the underlying processes or defects that lead them to have this disorder."[10]

- "There is a 100 percent increase per decade of life in the incidence of surgically managed pelvic organ prolapse in women from their 20's to their 70's."[11]

- "30 percent of women treated surgically for pelvic organ prolapse, urinary incontinence, or both will require re-operation for these processes."[12]

- "The more enlightened surgeons would tell their patients that the procedure would only last five years when it could be repeated as needed."[13]

- "The first surgical procedure performed is most likely to cure a patient's incontinence and have the fewest complications. Failure rates of subsequent procedures rise in proportion to the number of repeated procedures."[14]

- "Denervation [nerve damage] is recognized as a cause of female pelvic floor dysfunction, including urinary and fecal incontinence and pelvic relaxation."[15]

- "Anatomic and electrophysiologic studies have shown that the pudendal nerve and its branches play a central role in the innervation of the anal and urethral sphincters and other pelvic floor muscles."[16]

- "Pelvic floor damage can be reduced by minimizing forceps deliveries and episiotomies, by allowing passive decent in the second stage."[17]

- "The importance of neurological sequelae of vaginal surgery on the urethral sphincter and other pelvic floor muscles remains to be studied."[18]

- "Perhaps all that should be asked for is a set study that defines primary and secondary outcome variables while honestly reporting the side effects of those complications for the population undergoing the intervention."[19]

- "Recurrent pelvic organ prolapse is common and once a woman has undergone surgery for pelvic organ prolapse her risk of developing a further prolapse is 500 percent greater than in the general population."[20]

- "This implies a high rate of surgical failure. Although the reported surgical success rates based on small clinical populations exceed 90 percent, the true efficacy of these operations is unknown."[21]

- "Failure rates may be underestimated because success is often measured by the restoration of normal anatomy in a single compartment."[22]

- "It is said that new operations always work well 'for a while' with the originator of the operation always having the best success rates."[23]

- "Perhaps the concern we have with regard to pelvic floor defects is 'much ado about nothing'. On the other hand, one of our goals is to correct all anatomic defects, restore anatomy, and prevent recurrent vaginal support defects."[24]

- "All aspects of pelvic organ prolapse should be corrected simultaneously, even those that are mild or asymptomatic. However, this approach has never been prospectively demonstrated to correct or prevent more problems than it creates."[25]

- "It is with hope and anticipation that we look forward to exploring the new frontiers for pelvic floor disorders."[26]

Gynecologists have been studying the anatomy and physiology of the female pelvis for well over one hundred years. Their profound confusion over the cause of loss of pelvic organ support seems to run head-on into the central core of their practice, as illustrated in a symposium on the pelvic floor presented in the December 1966 issue of *Clinical Obstetrics & Gynecology*.[27] Dr. R. B. Durfee in his forward to that issue tells his fellow practitioners, "Pelvic organ support relies upon the preservation of interrelationships of pelvic tissue and the persistence of muscular response to pulsion in a complex system of checks and balances." He goes on to list the causes of pelvic organ prolapse: "But the major cause of pelvic tissue destruction is the stretching, dislocation, tearing, attenuation, and avulsion which occur in the pelvic tissues as a result of the passage of the fetal head during labor and delivery." He cautions, "The practice of exceedingly careful obstetrics, utilizing anesthesia and controlled early forceps delivery over an adequate prophylactic episiotomy will tend to obviate this damage. 'Push out,' spontaneous, or virtually unattended delivery are archaic from the standpoint of preventing trauma to the supportive structures of the pelvis. 'Ironing out the perineum' is an unacceptable practice from every stand point, but especially with regard to prophylactic preservation of genital tract supportive structures." Summing up the delicate problem for his fellows, he continues, "Since the universal practice of operative obstetrics and a reduction of the incidence of pelvic organ prolapse seems unlikely for some time to come, modern surgical methods must be applied to the repair of pelvic organ relaxation problems."

Durfee goes on to discuss the various surgical procedures for prolapse (the same ones in use today) and states, "There is an immediate restoration of function with amelioration of symptoms in 80 percent of patients treated by the majority of these methods. Unfortunately, there is a severely *decreasing* number of patients with *continued good results* as time passes... It would appear that the available tissues for use in plastic surgical procedures per vagina are frequently insufficient for permanent good results. Finally, far too often, the end result of extensive vaginoplasty is a rigid, tender, functionless, unyielding tube of tissue that is foreshortened and dry."† He concludes with the same sentiment expressed by our urogynecologists today that, "The broad field of corrective plastic gynecology" suggests "a future that is optimistic and stimulating."[28]

Nothing has changed since 1966, except for the numbers of women subjected to these operations. In 1997 in the United States, 226,210 women underwent 354,962 operations for prolapse[29] at a cost of 1 billion, 13 million dollars.[30] This does not include the number of operations performed strictly for urinary incontinence, nor does it reflect the number of hysterectomies done for other benign indications. Each year 600 thousand women are hysterectomized as the most common, non-pregnancy related surgery performed in the U.S.[31] It also leaves out the most hidden yet quite prevalent pelvic floor disorder—anal/rectal prolapse and fecal incontinence. These very common and often lifelong complications of third and fourth degree episiotomy wounds are most difficult to treat and cause untold suffering. A recent study found that all types of instrumental deliveries increased the risk of anal sphincter lacerations compared to spontaneous deliveries. Vacuum delivery increased the risk two-fold, and the risk was highest for forceps after an unsuccessful vacuum. Episiotomy significantly heightened the risk of anal sphincter damage, and compared to delivery by a general practitioner, delivery by an obstetrician increased the risk of sustaining a third or fourth degree laceration by 30 percent.[32]

In perhaps the most bizarre twist in the history of the medicalization of women's health, obstetricians, gynecologists, and urogynecologists are now urging women to consent to elective cesarean birth in order to protect the structures of the pelvic support system.[33] Young, healthy, uninformed mothers-to-be are presented with the Procrustean choice of vaginal childbirth that "May lead to severe damage of the pelvic floor and its component structures, with resultant negative effects"[34] or cesarean birth, "The only proven way that a woman can possibly protect her pelvic floor from the devastating effects of vaginal childbirth."[35] The irresponsibility of these statements is profound.

---

† *Emphasis in original*

With cesarean dissection (abdominal surgical birth), neonates are at risk for scalpel laceration, blunt intraabdominal injury, and respiratory complications.[36] Maternal risks include hemorrhage, infection, bowel paralysis, and pulmonary blood clot.[37] The rate of hysterectomy due to hemorrhage following cesarean birth is ten times greater than vaginal delivery, while the rate of maternal death increases sixteen-fold.[38] Mothers suffer the stress and pain of healing from major surgery, while at the same time having to continually lift and care for their newborn. Health care practitioners observe greater levels of frustration and self-doubt among these women than in women who have delivered vaginally. Long-term maternal complications following cesarean dissection are "frequently underestimated" and include the formation of adhesions, intestinal obstruction, and uterine scar dehiscence (rupture).[39] In addition, because of a recent, timesaving change in the way the uterus is sewn closed following cesarean delivery, women giving birth after a prior cesarean section are now at even greater risk of gross complication. For the past seventy-five years of routine cesarean delivery in the United States, the uterus has been closed using two layers of sutures.[40] It is now becoming common practice to place only one layer of sutures, leaving the muscle layer of the uterus to sometimes form a "window" of connective tissue instead of a durable scar.[41] This is now correlated with a dramatic rise in the incidence of an otherwise rare complication where the placenta adheres to the muscle wall of the uterus.[42] If there is only minimal adherence (placenta accreta), attempts at manual removal can be made, but if the adherence is severe (placenta percreta), maternal mortality rate from hemorrhage rises to 50 percent and hysterectomy is performed, as there is no other way to manage this obstetric emergency.

An observer commenting on soaring cesarean rates in Brazil (75 percent in some clinics) writes, "Medical practitioners have appropriated cultural values regarding the female body and sexuality, reinforced a blind fascination with technology, and medicalized women's fear of labor to justify their preference for surgical births."[43]

Drs. Abdul Sultan and Stuart Stanton reiterate, "As a result of this vicious circle of cultural phenomena and economic influences, enhanced by convenience for the obstetrician, cesarean section is becoming the most common delivery method in Brazil, while vaginal delivery is regarded as archaic, painful, disfiguring, and a cause of diminished sexual performance."[44] Furthermore, opening the pelvic cavity from above permanently damages nerves, disrupts fascial integrity, compromises the long-term health of the uterus, and has the potential to weaken the overall condition of the pelvic area, including the pelvic diaphragm. Cesarean deliveries presently comprise 25 percent of American births, and are steadily rising.

All reconstructive pelvic surgery puts the detrusor muscle, which wraps around the bladder, at risk of serious functional injury. Detrusor instability manifests as urge incontinence, or the inability to make it to the toilet in time after first sensing the need to urinate. This iatrogenic condition is known to occur following hysterectomy, vaginal dissection, and all incontinence surgeries. Urogynecologists continue to claim extremely high "cure" rates for stress incontinence, only to have inflicted a far more disabling condition, urge incontinence, on substantial percentages of their surgical populations.[45] The doctors are beginning to ask themselves the question, "Should a patient who is cured of stress incontinence and has refractory urge incontinence be considered cured? I think not, but I leave it to the individual reader to come to his or her own conclusion."[46]

It is difficult to come to terms with the fact that the (mostly) men in white coats who have treated us since adolescence belong to a club, a fraternity, an organization grounded in a nineteenth century machine model. Gynecology has formulated its own theories, devised its own experiments, and written its own rules. Even the surgeons debate the ethical quandary they find themselves in, richly illustrated in a recent issue of the *International Urogynecology Journal and Pelvic Floor Dysfunction*:

> *In the United States, the Food and Drug Administration (FDA) controls the introduction of new pharmaceutical agents into the marketplace. The FDA requires that new drugs are shown to be both safe and effective for the indications for which approval is sought before they are licensed for use in the United States. Most other industrialized nations have similar regulatory bodies. The ethical paradox is that although pharmacological innovation is tightly controlled by governmental regulation in most countries, surgical innovation is almost completely unregulated... New operations and new applications for older established operations may be introduced by individual surgeons without any controls establishing their validity, safety or effectiveness... There is no more powerful force in medicine than that of self-delusion.*[47]

Gynecology is a practice, not a scientific discipline. Medicine in general has very little to do with science. Rather, the practice of medicine is based on tradition, convention, and commerce, not hard scientific research. The medical system is a self-policing system. The certification of doctors is done by other doctors, and these people are not bound by such rigors of science as peer review, publication, and repeatable experiment.

Science itself suffers from the extreme limitations of a reductionist method of understanding reality. Reductionist reasoning focuses on parts of a system and attempts to deduce the whole from the sum of its parts. When reductionist reasoning is applied to the human body, as with many other vast systems, the complexities are virtually infinite, and whether or not all the parts are accounted for can never be fully ascertained. The renowned quantum physicist Vandana Shiva tells us that reductionist methodology "Has its uses in the fields of abstraction such as logic and mathematics, and in the fields of man-made artifacts such as mechanics. But it fails singularly to lead to a perception of reality (truth) in the case of living organisms such as nature, including man, in which the whole is not merely the sum of the parts, if only because the parts are so cohesively interrelated that isolating any part distorts perception of the whole." She goes on to explain that the entire way Western theory and practice have evolved is "The stuff of politics, not science. Picking one group of people (the specialists), who adopt one way of knowing the physical world (the reductionist), to find one set of properties in nature (the reductionist/mechanistic), is a political, not a scientific, act. It is this act that is claimed to be the 'scientific method.' The knowledge obtained is presented as the laws of nature—wholly 'objective' and altogether universal."[48]

The penetrating view of science has allowed many of the intricate workings of nature to be witnessed by us all. Who isn't completely awed by an electron-microscopic photograph of a germ being engulfed by a white blood cell, or a picture of some of the ten billion galaxies within range of our largest telescopes? The wonder of science is in its crystalline focus and immense depth. The problem with science is the extreme narrowness in how it looks at reality, with a piercing eye honed by exclusivity. This is why Western science has been largely unable to cure disease, save species, eradicate hunger, or improve the quality of life for most humans.

The materialistic-mechanistic-reductionist map is less than four centuries old, and parts of it, such as pelvic reconstructurive surgical theory, are much younger. Pelvic reconstructive surgery is a multibillion-dollar industry that focuses, as does much of Western medicine, on the relief of symptoms without addressing the underlying core issues of loss of pelvic organ support. Symptoms are the body's way of telling us things are out of balance. If we suppress or alter the symptom, the imbalance remains to create more severe symptoms and problems later on.

Women have been well trained to suppress their symptoms. They have also been frightened into complying with established methods of gynecologic treatment. Nowhere is this more prevalent than with the issue of cancer. Female reproductive organs are relentlessly referred to by practitioners as "potentially cancerous," "dangerous," and "unnecessary." The specter of cancer has persuaded generations of healthy women to part with their uteri and ovaries, only to subsequently suffer progressive pelvic system collapse and a multitude of other problems for which there are no solutions.

As with pelvic reconstructive surgery, it is time that the problem of cancer of the pelvic organs be thoroughly re-examined. The years following WWII saw the beginning of America's estrogen replacement therapy for women as well as the use of artificial estrogenic substances for such things as prevention of miscarriage. In 1955 it was observed that the rates of uterine and cervical malignancy had historically remained stable at a ratio of one to eight. In that same year a rapid rise in the occurence of uterine cancer was noted to be approaching a ratio of one to one.[49] It was during this same time period that women began taking "hormone shots."

The major hormonal factors involved in the development of uterine cancer have been recognized for decades, estrogen dominance being the only known cause of cancer of the lining of the uterus.[50] Nutritional deficiency is now understood to be a major reason the cervix succumbs to pathologic cell changes incited primarily by viruses.[51] However, this knowledge has yet to be integrated into a holistic, general understanding of total pelvic health.†

Re-search means to look again. The Western medical model is built upon a mechanistic map completely outmoded by physics and the life sciences. Four hundred years of dissection and more than one hundred years of pelvic reconstructive surgery illustrate that a machine cannot change, grow, or evolve. A new energy must now create a spiral out of the endless circle chase of disease and destruction to women.

As science returns to an ancient, organic concept of the universe, medicine must also strive to better understand nature's inner harmonies, symmetries, and proportions. We have seen that we wander afield of nature at our own peril and, to quote a nuclear physicist speaking recently on National Public Radio, "It is Mother Nature's job to make fools out of scientists." Each part of nature's design has a place and function, all working together to serve in ways we have yet begun to understand. The woman who learns to listen to and trust in her body's capacity to return to wholeness is creating the very stuff of her own growth and evolution. For the energy that creates a spiral out of a circle is the energy of life itself.

∾

---

† *Because progestins have been combined with estrogen in hormone replacement therapy, these preparations lower the risk of endometrial cancer than in previous decades, but still highten the risk of breast cancer, ovarian cancer, and cardiovascular disease particularly stroke.*

Pregnancy & Prolapse

"If the basic needs of labouring women had been understood, we would not already be the witnesses of the second or third generation of high-tech childbirth"

MICHEL ODENT
The Caesarean[1]

PELVIC ORGAN PROLAPSE DURING AND AFTER PREGNANCY has affected women down through the ages. It happens to sheep, cows, horses, zoo animals, and the occasional animal in the wild. Farmers know about pregnancy and prolapse as do race horse owners, veterinarians, and naturalists. The only place there seems to be a knowledge-vacuum on the subject is in the field of obstetrics and gynecology: "A key-word search of 'uterine prolapse,' 'uterovaginal prolapse,' or 'procidentia' with 'pregnancy' was conducted on Medline and very few references were found, especially in the past decade."[2]

A uterine prolapse that presents during pregnancy is perhaps the most frightening. Not only is there the initial shock and dread of an externalized organ, but also fear for the well-being of a seemingly displaced fetus. "I cannot believe how much this prolapse has affected me", Nicola writes. "I've been totally consumed by it and worried my stress will rub off on my beautiful unborn child."

Nicola's doctor told her not to worry, that her cervix would rise back up by the beginning of the second trimester, and that her symptoms would probably not return. Although it is unusual for the prenatal cervix to reach all the way to the introitus, current studies demonstrate that prolapse is very common during pregnancy. In a large study of pregnant American soldiers nearly half were diagnosed with stage two pelvic organ prolapse.[3] Nicola's symptoms did resolve, but her lingering questions remained: "Should I have a cesarean? Will a vaginal delivery cause the prolapse to return?" Her answers would not be easily forthcoming.

Severe prenatal prolapse may be relatively uncommon, but postpartum prolapse seems to be occurring in epidemic numbers. Although prolapse develops after gentle home births and c-sections, the vast majority of postpartum symptoms follow common

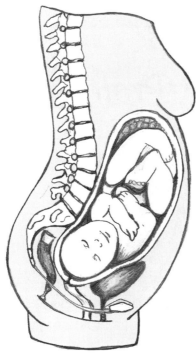

Figure 6-1
Maternal Pelvis

obstetric interventions. Many studies during the past decade have correlated routine use of such practices as epidural analgesia, episiotomy, vacuum extraction, and forceps with maternal vaginal injury. Giving birth while restrained in the lithotomy position narrows the pelvic outlet and causes undue pressure and stretching of soft tissue structures[4]

Maternal injury is considered by much of the medical establishment to be an inevitable outcome of vaginal delivery and demonstrably little effort has been made to separate truly natural birth from interventionist hospital strategies when considering outcomes. Given the perplexing attitude that "all vaginal births are created equal" it is no wonder many practitioners are calling for cesarean section as a preventive measure to protect against maternal vaginal injury. However easily obstetricians and gynecologists may be swayed toward sanctioning elective c-section, cutting through the musculature of the lower abdominal wall, dissecting the uterus off its attachments to the bladder, and then lifting the uterus out of the mother's body in order to repair it with permanent sutures, yields anything but prevention from prolapse and incontinence.[5,6] It has been estimated that seven to nine women would have to deliver by cesarean to prevent one woman from having a disorder of pelvic organ support.[7,8]

Probable causes involved in the development of postpartum prolapse include soft tissue damage and skeletal misalignment. During labor and delivery the vaginal walls are pulled and stretched from basement layers of tissue connecting them to surrounding structures. This stretching and avulsing is well documented and undisputed by doctors and women alike. However, rarely does a woman stand up after giving birth to realize her bladder and bowel have prolapsed into her vagina. Far more frequently, it is two or more weeks postpartum before her symptoms show up. This is very interesting. If soft tissue injury from the birth process itself was the primary cause of postpartum prolapse, would the damage not present itself immediately?

Answers to that enigma may lie in the mechanics of the birth process itself (Figure 6-1). Recall in the Pelvic Organ Support chapter we learned about the concept of sacral nutation. This ability of the sacrum to rock forward and backward on the hipbones is essen-

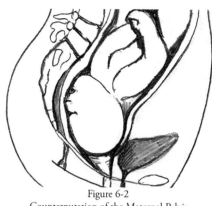

Figure 6-2
Counternutation of the Maternal Pelvis

tial for opening the birth canal so the baby can pass through. In the non-pregnant state, the sacrum is doing this slight rocking back and forth motion throughout the day as we move about. However, during the last two-to-three weeks of pregnancy the baby drops into the top of the bony birth canal. This is called "lightening" and is usually accompanied by more freedom in the upper abdomen and chest, and therefore easier breathing. In order for the baby to have room to move into the lower part of the pelvis, the sacrum must move out. It does this by rocking back into the counternutated position where it stays until the baby is born (Figure 6-2). The maternal lumbar curve flattens in advanced pregnancy.[9] During the second stage of labor after the baby's head and shoulders have navigated the front of the pelvis, the sacrum rocks forward and the tailbone lifts up to make room for the baby to traverse the back of the pelvis (Figure 6-3). This is the reason it is so important to have the back of the pelvis able to move freely during the birth process.

It is a reasonable question to ask, "What are the consequences of the spine being set for weeks in the counternutated position?" Not the slightest reference to this matter is to be found anywhere in pregnancy, obstetric, gynecologic, or orthopedic literature. Therefore, we can only wonder whether there may be some relationship between the counternutated maternal spine and the development of pelvic organ prolapse in the weeks following delivery. If the number of new mothers developing the very common postpartum cystocele/rectocele has remained unchanged over the centuries, would not more women know about it? Would there not exist folklore, anecdotes, wives tales, and ancient medical advice for such a common malady? "Fallen womb" is a very old and fairly common literary reference. Yet, the terms we use for postpartum cystocele and rectocele have their origin in medical language as does the word "prolapse."

Young mothers are highly valued members of all societies. Perhaps if prolapse information has been lost in our own culture, there are others that speak of such common disorders affecting postpartum women. Yet,

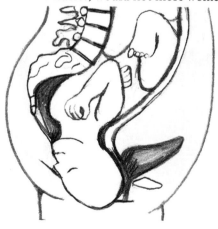

Figure 6-3
Nutation of Maternal Pelvis

not even a faint whisper on the subject echoes from the halls of anthropology.

Well then, can the type of postpartum vaginal wall collapse that develops a few weeks after delivery be a new disorder? And if so, could it be related to the same amount of time the maternal spine spends in counternutation before labor even begins? What has changed to cause such an epidemic of prolapse in the postpartum population?

These are questions worthy of humanity's interest. In the meantime, it is a logical theory based in scientific fact that pelvic tissues are unwound in the weeks before delivery due to the counternutated position of the pelvis. Add to this the effect of pregnancy hormones relaxing pelvic joints for maximum flexibility and it becomes clear the inherent musculoskeletal stability of the human female in advanced pregnancy is compromised. Yet, this is the way the biomechanics of pregnancy have worked down through the ages and every human society understands the special need of the gravid woman to be sheltered.

What *is* different is that modern women are no longer restoring the natural curvature to their spine in the weeks following birth. Largely because of helpful husbands, convenience foods, upholstered furniture, and labor-saving devices, many maternal spines remain in flexion throughout much of the day as mothers recline and spend time with their newborn. In olden times, women resumed their work load in the days and weeks following delivery, which by its very nature restored spinal shape, vaginal axis, and pelvic organ placement in the new mother. Rest and posture are equally important.

What we do know for certain, whether prolapse results from a gentle home birth or an instrumental delivery, it is a devastating experience to feel as if your bottom is going to drop out at any moment. Jane describes the experience well:

> *Discovering prolapse was difficult for me. So much so that even the thought of my daughter's birthday (I discovered prolapse shortly after her birth) made fear rise up in me. I was so angry and devastated and trying to deal with a newborn on top of that. Standing and especially holding her while standing made the falling out feeling much worse. I felt like a terrible mother and I hated what had happened to my body.*

As with prolapse at any age, postpartum prolapse in the young woman is responded to by medical doctors in narrowly defined, predictable ways. "My GP gave me no information whatsoever about my prolapse and I had to dig deeper myself to find out what it was she was referring me to a specialist for," Michelle tells us. "She talked about vaginal hysterectomy before I even knew what it was I was truly diagnosed with." Anna received a similar response, "My prolapse occurred about three to four weeks after the birth of my third child. Then I waited for my postpartum appointment with my doctor. It was hard to accept the reality. I had cried for weeks. I was urged to undergo the surgery. The doctor told me to stop breastfeeding then wait three to four months and set up surgery." Six weeks after an instrumental delivery, Sandy returned to her doctor, "It was my bladder out of position and he mentioned surgery immediately. I was freaked out."

Unlike their obedient mothers and grandmothers, women of today are quicker to question authority. Ann tells us, "When my obstetrician looked me in the eye and said, 'You will have surgery at some point in your lifetime' I really felt like she had no right to make that assertion and that I need to release that 'sentence' from my body."

At no time in history have we had better insight into the way prolapsed women are treated by medical science. "My doctor told me the same thing, well worse" says Beth. "He said I would need a hysterectomy eventually. My uterus hadn't even prolapsed!" "Both of the doctors I saw recommended hysterectomy" Maya added. "I'm 32 years old!"

Radical pelvic surgery is not the only medical treatment commonly offered to postpartum mothers. "I recently had my second son and at my postpartum checkup I found out that I have a prolapsed uterus. I am totally freaked out about it," Tanya tells us. "My doctor says that it may be due to low levels of estrogen since I'm breastfeeding and prescribed Premarin cream to use at night. She says it may fix itself with the cream." At six weeks postpartum Brenda was told by her doctor that if her cystocele did not resolve in three months, "He could do surgery. I'm also on the Estrace cream once a week." "My doctor prescribed the same thing," says Rachael. "I have the tube sitting upstairs in my bathroom. So far I haven't used it because I'm breast feeding and wary of the estrogen getting into my breast milk, although my son's pediatrician assures me it's not a problem."

Beyond dangerous drugs, surgery, and the occasional pessary fitting, the medical community does not know what to do about prolapse and therefore has been highly resistant to change. But change it must because the traditional response to the newly prolapsed woman is no longer acceptable or appropriate by any standard of measure.

As for postpartum prolapsed women, there is great reason for optimism. Women are, as Jane says, "Learning to deal with what was once devastating news and learning that it is a livable situation that does get better with time." Lysa, just five weeks postpartum, tells us, "My bladder was right at the opening and now it's back to normal 95 percent of the time. I can't feel my cervix most of the time and it was just about on the outside and the rectocele behaves unless I don't watch my diet."

Obstetricians and gynecologists have long been aware of the prevalence of maternal injury sustained in childbirth. However, few public health statistics exist on the subject, and doctors have traditionally expressed little interest in studying how postpartum prolapse might be reduced. A thorough, if not widely known, discussion on maternal vaginal injury was presented in the 1989 classic, *Vaginal Surgery,* by highly esteemed pelvic reconstructive surgeons, David Nichols and Clyde Randall.[10] Yet, little more appeared in medical literature on making vaginal birth safer for women. The authors begin with the statement,

> *In the annals of medical and surgical literature, the reviewer expects to find record of cumulative knowledge which has been responsible for improving the effectiveness of treatment. In the practice of obstetrics and gynecology during the 20th century, however, preventative measures have proven to be most effective.*

Their words hold just as true today as surgeons continue to perform the same defective operations and women continue to experience the same disastrous results. Drs. Clyde and Randall continue their commentary with even stronger charges:

Stated most simply, there seems to have been a lack of interest or documentation indicating study of the manner in which human parturition can be managed so the effectiveness of preventative measures has been generally recognized, obstetric practices seem to have neglected opportunities to initiate more effective efforts to lessen the maternal injury and subsequent disability possible and not infrequently attributable to the conduct of childbirth. It would seem as though there has been a rather general acceptance of the probability of injury and the need for subsequent repair of maternal tissues as unavoidable consequences of human parturition. During the years while surgical repair of varying types and degrees of maternal injury has been thoroughly described, relatively little has been spoken or written to suggest techniques and procedures recommended to reduce the frequency and extent of maternal injuries.

These authors asked the same perplexing question in 1989 that women are still agonizing over today:

Is the occurrence of genital dysfunction due to maternal injury and the discomfort women experience because of pelvic relaxation of little or no concern to the obstetrician? Is the obstetrician-gynecologist justified in concluding 'If it bothers her we can certainly do a satisfactory repair whenever she wants it done?' Such a willingness to disregard the possible effectiveness of prophylactic measures would not seem compatible with usual professional points of view. We believe there are indeed other factors that have accounted for the undeniable fact that the 'teachers' of obstetric practice at the undergraduate, graduate, and continuing education levels have, for the most part, failed to emphasize how labor and delivery can best be managed in order to avoid or minimize maternal tissue damage. For generations dedicated teachers of obstetrics have emphasized and personally practiced conservative obstetrics. A virtually universal willingness to perpetuate the conviction that 'nature does it best' has made certain that each medical student and resident-in-training becomes sufficiently experienced in the observation of spontaneous delivery that they will recognize and remember the factors accounting for the abilities of the female to deliver normally, while at the same time appreciating the satisfaction of the 'natural' delivery of a normal child.

As practicing obstetrician-gynecologists, Nichols and Randall became acutely interested in "Why prolapse later in some patients and not in so many others who were presumably exposed to the same forces of labor and delivery?" They were not to be persuaded by the argument that congenital predisposition to weak connective tissue accounts for most cases of prolapse because "In a majority of instances only the trauma of labor and delivery seems to suggest an etiology." Careful examination revealed that rather than weak tissue being unable to support the birthing process, it is often strong tissue offering resistance to the dynamics of labor that cause the majority of maternal injury.

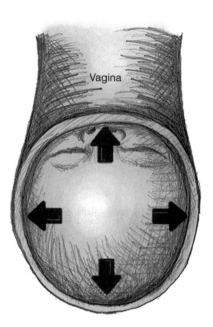

Vagina

Figure 6-4
Formation of Distension Cystocele

Nichols and Randall observed that most birthing women do not have the urge to bear down with their contractions until the fetal head (or breech) begins to distend the pubococcygeus muscle. By this time the cervix is fully dilated and the presenting part can easily descend into the vagina with the force of contractions. The doctors gave very clear warnings of the damage most likely to occur if a woman were coached to push too early:

When such premature bearing down does occur, certainly the tissues supporting both the fundus and the cervix in normal anatomic relationships with the bony pelvis and adjacent viscera must either succeed in resisting the woman's efforts to 'deliver her uterus with the baby in it' or her efforts will result in considerably more stretching and detachment of uterine supporting tissues than would have occurred had there been no bearing down effort before the cervix was fully dilated.

Precipitous pushing is an obvious cause of tissue damage, as is the simple geometry of a large fetus leaving the vaginal walls "stretched beyond the ability of tone-regaining involuntary processes to restore to a non-redundant caliber." It is worth noting, however, that midwives the world over speak of the enormous capacity of vaginal tissue to stretch without noticeable damage. Yet, harm to the elasticity and integrity of the vaginal wall itself remains one possible type of injury noted by these authors. As we learned in chapter 4, Surgical Intervention, distention cystocele results from overstretching of the vagina itself and is believed to be related in some cases to long labor and pressure necrosis. Occasionally a short, precipitous labor where distension is so rapid that vaginal muscle cells do not have time to adapt may also cause this sort of prolapse (Figure 6-4). Displacement cystocele is thought to occur when the vagina becomes stretched and detached from the supporting tissues underneath that keep it anchored in its proper position within the pelvis (Figure 6-5). Further study by Nichols and Randall revealed striking and important information as to the probable cause of much of the damage resulting in postpartum cystocele, rectocele, and uterine prolapse:

To understand and anticipate vaginal injuries commonly associated with parturition, the attendants should recognize that normally, and certainly in the labor of the primapara [first-time mother], *at full dilation of the cervix the presenting part does not at that time emerge from the cervix and, for the first time, begin to descend into and through the vagina. Rather, the fully engaged presenting part, almost completely covered by thinned, beginning to dilate cervix, has in all probability occupied the upper third to half of the vagina for 2 or more weeks. As a result, distention of the upper vagina, with accommodation of the engaging vertex or breech, has occurred very gradually, so gradually in fact that the patient may not be aware of the descent taking place until she notices a new awareness of heaviness, low backache, and at times rectal pressure, while at the same time breathing becomes somewhat easier, for "lightening" has occurred.*

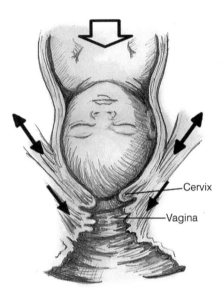

Figure 6-5
Formation of Displacement Cystocele

However, the researchers found that such is not always the case, especially with the multigravida, or woman who is giving birth for the second or more time, and who experiences a short, intense labor. Gradual distention may not occur before the fetus begins to descend rapidly through an undilated upper vagina. Likewise, if the first-time mother begins labor with the presenting part not engaged, her vaginal tissues become vulnerable to injury even if they are very strong.

Nichols and Randall note that "Under such circumstances the force of uterine contractions may tend to push an undulating, contraction ring-like segment of vagina ahead of the presenting part. If this situation persists the forces of labor will be exerted, not so much on distending or dilating the vagina as upon the supporting fascia that is trying to hold that segment of vagina in its normal position within the maternal pelvis."

With each contraction, the forces that are pushing the fetus down the vaginal canal begin to push a fold of vagina ahead of the presenting part, pulling on the fascial fibers underneath the undilated segment of vaginal wall (Figure 6-6).

Under such circumstances, descent can be accomplished only by pushing the undilated segment or ring of vaginal wall ahead of the presenting part. In all probability, once a resisting contraction ring-like segment of vagina is pushed ahead of the presenting part, the damage to vaginal supporting tissue has been done. As the fascial attachments give way, the rim or roll of resisting, undilated vaginal wall irons out rapidly, and descent of the presenting part proceeds to the perineal stage. There is no evidence of the damage done until weeks later when postpartum examination reveals loss of vaginal rugae and a loss of the concavity of the superior vaginal fornices. The persistence of redundant vaginal wall and the development of eversion (with or without uterine prolapse) confirm that a satisfactory reattachment of vaginal wall support does not necessarily occur spontaneously during involutionary tightening of the pelvic fascial planes.

Nichols and Randall became keen researchers into the process of vaginal injury and contributed vital information on how to avoid the most common types of maternal soft tissue damage as a result of labor and delivery. Their primary recommendations were to encourage relaxation so that the upper vagina may fully dilate; to never coach a birthing woman to bear down with contractions until the cervix is known to be fully dilated; and not until the presenting part has come down through the upper vagina and is beginning to distend the perineum.

In keeping with the philosophical framework of their profession, Nichols and Randall advised implementation of their recommendations through total obstetric management of labor, including use of anesthesia, oxytocic hormones, episiotomy, and forceps. A decade later when it became obvious that this level of intervention was only increasing maternal soft tissue damage, the American College of Obstetricians and Gynecologists began to promote elective cesarean as a preventive measure against vaginal injury and pelvic floor dysfunction.

The midwifery model of care recognizes the profound importance of relaxation to the process of natural childbirth. Ina May Gaskin writes about "sphincter law" and the role maternal emotions play in the healthy progression of labor.[11] Obstetrician-midwife Michel Odent is the world's leading advocate of a "wise maternal figure" being present with the birthing mother. Several studies have shown that this type of attendant is most associated with calming maternal anxiety and producing healthy birth outcomes.[12] Unfamiliar surroundings of hospital and staff are believed by many educators to be primarily responsible for the psychological barrier associated with obstructed labor. Furthermore, the majority of birthing women requesting anesthesia do so believing labor will be more relaxed and comfortable if sedated. Childbirth researcher Penny Simkin tells us,

Normally, the woman's pelvic floor provides a resilient platform on which the fetal head

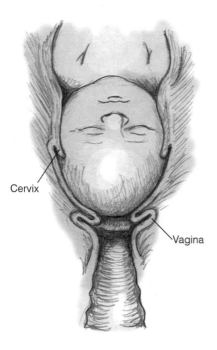

Figure 6-6
Formation of Vaginal Wall Injury

Cervix

Vagina

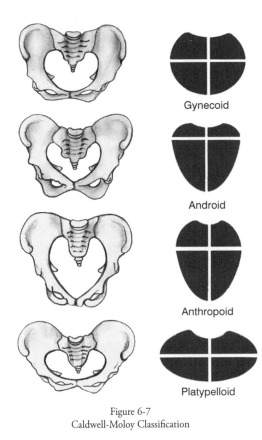

Figure 6-7
Caldwell-Moloy Classification

Gynecoid

Android

Anthropoid

Platypelloid

can rotate, and the muscles lining the pelvis also provide a resilient cushion that encourages rotation. Pressure on these muscles elicits a stretch response that plays an important role in the cardinal movements of descent (flexion, internal rotation, extension, and external rotation). However, when anesthetized, there is a reduction in the tone of these muscles, which tends to inhibit rotation of the fetal head. When combined with maximal breath-holding and straining by the woman, the likelihood of persistent malposition or a deep transverse arrest is greatly increased. [13]

Through extensive study, Nichols and Randall concluded that the majority of maternal injuries sustained during vaginal delivery are not the result of genetic weakness, but ensue from the mechanical forces of the birth process. No consideration of the dynamics of childbirth would be complete without careful focus on the bony birth passage itself. The evolution of the human pelvis culminated in a design perfectly balanced between bipedal efficiency and birthing capacity.

The primate birth canal is essentially a straight, horizontal tube with a sacrum that lacks the broad concavity marking the human sacrum. Even in our closest hominid relatives, the pelvic inlet and outlet are situated along the same geometric plane, while in humans the long axes of the openings are perpendicular. This results in a curvature to the birth passage that requires the fetus to make several complex maneuvers over the course

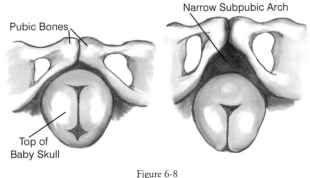

Pubic Bones

Narrow Subpubic Arch

Top of
Baby Skull

Figure 6-8
Subpubic Arch

of delivery.[14]

During the 1930s, obstetricians Caldwell and Moloy believed they had identified four distinct human female pelvic shapes, (Figure 6-7) a classification scheme that can still be found in obstetric textbooks today. Not without racial overtones, this typing system also has proven less than accurate in predicting what ethnic group of women might possess a particularly shaped pelvis. It is now understood that the rounded, anatomically superior "gynecoid" pelvic shape appears in about half of all women, regardless of race or ethnicity. Furthermore, the shape of the female pelvis is considered to have more to do with developmental factors than genetic inheritance.[15]

While cephalo-pelvic disproportion is a rare occurrence and the vast majority of women are able to birth vaginally if given proper support, pelvic shape can be a determining factor in the development of some forms of prolapse. If the subpubic arch is more "android" or narrow (a relatively uncommon finding), the fetal skull must move back against the posterior vaginal wall to be born (Figure 6-8). This could possibly cause inordinate stretching of the back vaginal wall and lead to future rectocele, especially if delivering in the lithotomy position. Since the process of human birth moves the fetus down and back from the abdominal wall, maternal birthing postures that best facilitate this dynamic should be encouraged.

The important observations of maternal injury made almost two decades ago by Nichols and Randall have yet to be validated by other teams of researchers. The obvious worth of the subject matter cannot be overemphasized; it is a disgrace so few studies exist on maternal injury and prenatal and postpartum prolapse.

Nevertheless, except in extreme cases, symptoms of postpartum prolapse are similar regardless of method of vaginal delivery. It is also true that once women begin to strengthen the natural shape of their spine, symptoms begin to improve. The Whole Woman™ Posture is also ideal for another very common postpartum condition, diastasis recti, where the normal separation in the rectus abdominus muscles has widened around the navel area. Pulling the abdomen *up* instead of *in* causes tightening along natural fascial planes and a drawing together of the recti toward the center.

Women healing naturally from prolapse often begin to realize a deepening femininity and stronger sense of self. Marie describes it beautifully: "Due to prolapse, I have cultivated much more awareness of my femaleness and comfort with my body! I feel more feminine and beautiful. I wear different clothes. Prettier, more flowing, less restrictive... It's the way I hold myself now, too... I hold my head proudly. I'm more connected to my whole self."

❧

Lighting the Lamp

THE REASON SO LITTLE PROGRESS HAS BEEN MADE in the treatment of prolapse and incontinence is because generations of doctors, nurses, physical therapists and women have been taught to look at the problem as if the world were flat. *One* dimension of *one* structure within the female pelvis has been the primary focus of surgical and nonsurgical treatments for over a century. A recent story illuminates the level of pain and suffering women have endured from the one-dimensional world of reconstructive pelvic surgery.

In 2002 Leslie was given the "gold standard" treatment for stage 3 uterine prolapse. At age forty-three she underwent uterosacrocolpopexy, posterior colporrhaphy, and retropubic bladder neck suspension. By 2003 she was diagnosed with stage 3 prolapse of the uterus and back vaginal wall, and after two years of suffering severe symptoms, consented in December of 2005 to a sub-total hysterectomy and second sacrocolpopexy. By the fall of 2006 Leslie was in constant pain from the total collapse of her vaginal vault. Upon returning to the same well-known and highly regarded urogynecology group for evaluation, she was told her cervix would now need to be removed but that her vaginal walls were well-supported. When asked, "What, then, is the large, obstructive bulge at the back of my vagina and what's to be done about the unrelenting pressure at my perineum?", her doctor replied, "Oh, that can be fixed by Kegels."

Kegels, or pelvic wall contractions, have been not only the gold standard, but the sole standard of nonsurgical treatment for all conditions of pelvic organ support. Like pumping biceps or quads, contractions of the pelvic wall are believed to strengthen the levator ani, build up support for the urethra, and reposition prolapsed organs. Even though these thin, sinewy rings of muscle are capable of very little movement and act primarily as stabilizers of the bony pelvis and compressors of the external sphincters.

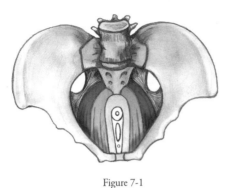

Figure 7-1
Frontal View of Female Pelvis in Standing Position

Concentric rings of muscle extend from the pubic bones to behind the anus and rectum, to connect onto the tailbone (Figure 7-1). A contraction of these horseshoe-shaped muscles draws the anus, vagina, and urethra forward toward the pubic bones. During urination and defecation, we relax these muscles so that the sphincters will open. Upon completion, the muscles automatically contract and pull forward, expelling the final portion of urine or feces. This important function makes elimination as clean and efficient as possible. This is what the pelvic wall muscles do. They are better adapted to helping things go out than keeping things in. For keeping organs and bodily fluids in we have several other highly specialized mechanisms such as the biaxial pelvis, complex internal and external sphincters, and when all else fails, squeezing together the buttocks and muscles of the thigh.

The so-called pelvic wall has two functions when it contracts: reinforcing the pelvic sphincters like the coming together of a pair of elevator doors, and pulling forward on the pubic bones to complete elimination. Ancillary functions include dropping the tailbone, which results in the counternutation of the sacrum required for many movements including walking, sitting, lying down, and giving birth; and relaxing to initiate evacuation of bladder and bowels.

All physical therapy for prolapse and incontinence is focused not only on the pelvic wall, but on one dimension of the pelvic wall. The long Y-axis from pubic bone to tailbone is the focus of Kegels. By contracting several times a day along the Y-axis something is supposed to happen. Yet, generations of women are still waiting to find out what. This is because the Y-axis has very little involvement in pelvic organ support.

However, women begin stabilizing and reversing the symptoms of prolapse and incontinence when they learn that the pelvic outlet has another dimension. The X-axis runs across the diameter of the pelvic wall from ischial spine to ischial spine. A strong, fascia-wrapped layer of horizontal muscle is fused underneath the front half of the pelvic wall. This muscle, the deep perineal muscle, does not contract on its own, but follows the movement of the sides of the pubic bone it is attached to.

Add the all-important third dimension, weight-loading from above, and the pelvic wall tightens like a drum (Figure 7-2). As the tailbone lifts, the muscles are stretched along their long Y-axis. As the sit bones and posterior aspect of the pubic bones widen, the X-axis expands, stretching taut from one pelvic sidewall to the other. Because the urethra is embedded in the X-axis, it is raised and supported in its anatomical position only when the X-axis tightens. In this position it is lifted into the physiologic pelvis where it receives the same amount of intraabdominal pressure the bladder does, so that continence is maintained.

The people who brought us Kegels actually had it backwards. Contracting the Y-axis plays a primary role in elimination. Lengthening the Y-axis creates the necessary conditions for pelvic organ support and urinary continence. Barbaric treatments such as intravaginal electrical stimulation (e-stim) target only one dimension of muscle activity, the Y-axis, with no regard for the three-dimensional anatomy of pelvic organ support.

The urinary continence system is a well protected, highly stable mechanism. Barring severe trauma it is even responsive to contractions of the pelvic wall, which move it forward along the Y-axis. Yet repetitive

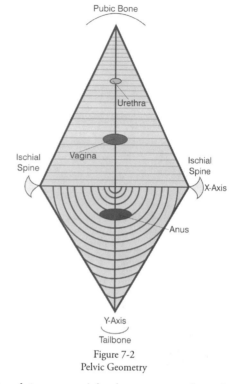

Figure 7-2
Pelvic Geometry

Kegels performed with a flexed spine, such as when lying on one's back, may strain the tailbone area and aggravate a cystocele by pulling the bladder away from the lower abdominal wall. A much more effective way to perform perineal contractions for prolapse and/or incontinence is to position yourself in a right angle seated posture with your lumbar curve in place. This way all the muscles of the perineum are strengthened while your urethra is lifted into its proper physiologic position.

Movement of the bony pelvis itself controls and orchestrates the mass action of muscles that tighten and lock the pelvic organs into position. The pelvic wall is like a drum skin through which the urethra, vagina, and rectum pass. When the drum is tight these channels are elevated, well-supported, and in their functional positions. When the drum is loose, as it is when the tailbone is flexed, these structures become less supported. When we spend our lives in spinal flexion, as most women in the modern world do, conditions for prolapse and incontinence become ripe, as the soft-tissue structures of birth and elimination lose strength, elasticity, and their inherent form and function. Pelvic organs become subject to being blown out of the body instead of pinned into place by the forces of intra-abdominal pressure. Women then turn to doctors, who practice surgeries founded upon gross anatomical error.

Andreas Vesalius (1514-1564) was a Flemish anatomist and medical artist who worked for the most influential surgeons of his time. The Vesalius drawings of the human

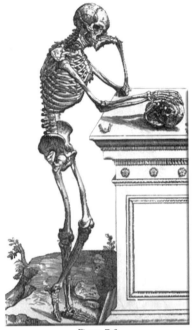

Figure 7-3
Vesalius's Incorrect Pelvic Orientation

pelvis became the universally accepted medical interpretation of pelvic orientation (Figure 7-3). However, because he created his spinal model by mounting the vertebrae on a vertical iron rod, the sacral curvature was lost and the orientation of the rest of the pelvis distorted. This was the beginning of visualizing and illustrating the human pelvis as a "bowl" with a "floor" and pelvic organs precariously perched in a "hammock" spanning horizontally from pubic bone to tailbone (Figure 7-4).

Such a quaint error in judgment is certainly understandable as early scientific medical men struggled with the anatomy of their subject matter. What is incomprehensible is that the misrepresentation continues to this day. In 1993 two professors of veterinary medicine from Purdue University tried to draw professional attention to the issue. "A persistent error in many anatomical textbooks used today presents a modified inferior view of the pelvis as the 'front view' and a nearly accurate front view as a 'view from above'. No definitive conclusion can be reached concerning the reason(s) for the remarkably long persistence of this error."[2]

While we can be grateful to the veterinarians for politely pointing out the mistake, the problem of the misrepresented pelvis was convincingly argued in the gynecologic literature by J. W. Davies in 1954.[3] Regrettably, his artful and original presentation caused not a ripple of effect as journals and textbooks continued to portray the female pelvis with a full 45-degree positional inaccuracy. The pubic bone is consistently drawn where the mons pubis (the mound of flesh and hair below the navel) would be, or higher, and on

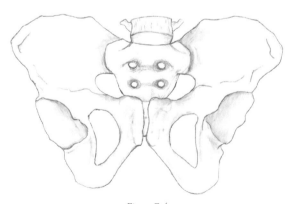

Figure 7-4
Incorrect Position of Pelvis

a horizontal plane with the coccyx. A concave soft tissue floor is often shown with dramatic representation of how easy nature has made it for pelvic organs to fall out of such an arrangement (Figure 7-5).

In their comprehensive surgical text *The Female Pelvic Floor,* Linda Brubaker and Theodore Sacclarides took the opportunity to enlighten their colleagues about the age-old error and clearly illustrate the cor-

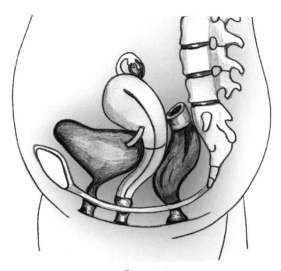

Figure 7-5
Common Anatomical Error

rect position of the pelvis. Using the original Davies schematics (Figure 7-6 A & B), these authors pointed out that if the human pelvis was actually positioned like a bowl (Figure 7-6B), walking would not only be excruciatingly painful, but impossible, because the pubic symphysis would immediately dislocate.[4] The issue is settled and we learn about the pubic bones as they truly exist, like the straps of a saddle coming together directly underneath the torso and between the legs. Yet, these same authors allow sketch after sketch throughout the rest of the

book to represent the position of the pelvis in archaic Vesalius inaccuracy.

Far more disturbing are published photographs of x-rays of the female pelvis supposedly taken from the side view in standing posture. These are likely embalmed cadavers that have been radiographed and then "stood up" in the illustration. The most nimble of contortionists could not stand up with her pelvis in the Vesalius position. We now move beyond ignorance, for it would take deceit to portray an x-ray of a 45-degree pelvic rotation in the standing position. Embarrassing at best are recent attempts at building elaborate biomechanical models of prolapse based on inaccurate anatomy.

The implications of surgical techniques and procedures that begin with an inaccurate understanding of the surrounding bone structure are staggering. Reconstructive pelvic surgery patients are often placed in Trendelenburg position, on their back with the head of the surgical table slightly

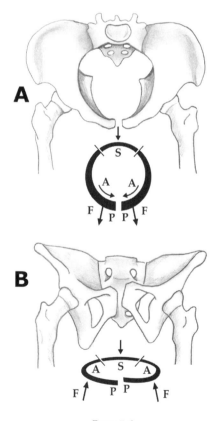

Figure 7-6
A: Correct & B: Incorrect Pelvic Orientation

lowered. Their hips are then rotated backward and their legs positioned up and out to the sides in stirrups. This position carries significant risk of pelvic and lower limb nerve injury and also the potentially catastrophic compartment syndrome that results from low blood pressure in the lower extremity. "It has been estimated that the fall in lower limb pressure is 2mmHg for every vertical inch in height of the leg above the heart."[5]

Beyond the acute risks of surgical lithotomy is the astonishing irony that the degree of posterior hip rotation required of the position places the pelvis in precisely the same plane relative to the rest of the spine as the Vesalius drawings! There is now a "floor" through which the pelvic interior is entered. In this position the organs are pulled by the gravity of their weight away from the abdominal wall and opposite that of natural standing posture, while anesthesia totally relaxes voluntary and involuntary muscle alike. It is in this position that pelvic organs, ligaments, and fascia are cut, pulled, sutured, and stapled to the surrounding bone structure.

When these women once again resume standing posture, *they do so with a pelvic interior reconstructed around a 45-degree backward rotation*. Women, in their own words, describe the pain of living in a body struggling to reconfigure around twisted anatomy.

- "At times the pain is so bad I can't find a comfortable position or anything that will relieve it."

- "The mesh is eroding more and more. I can feel it in my vagina and it's irritating me all the time. The blue color of the mesh even shows through my skin. My urogynecologist told me that leaving the mesh in is not going to hurt me."

- "I've had eight treatments with silver nitrate for granulation tissue overlying the exposed mesh. None of the doctors I've seen are willing to try to remove it."

- "I had a cystocele and rectocele repair six months ago. I have problems with bowel movements still and the pressure and heaviness are unbearable. My urogynecologist said that I was fine and that all women have rectoceles and that was it."

- "I don't know where to turn and I'm scared."

The world is round. The form and function of normal female pelvic anatomy cannot be recreated through surgery. Pelvic organ support depends upon seven aspects of a three-dimensional reality grounded in natural posture and movement:

- Natural breathing
- Force of intra-abdominal pressure
- Biaxial shape of the female torso
- Biaxial positions of the pelvic organs
- A fully intact perineal body
- Internal resting pressure of the urethra
- X and Y axes of the pelvic wall.

∾

part two
Restoring Our Natural Design

In the beginner's mind
there are many possibilities,
but in the expert's there are
few.

SHUNRYU SUZUKI
Zen Mind,
Beginner's Mind[1]

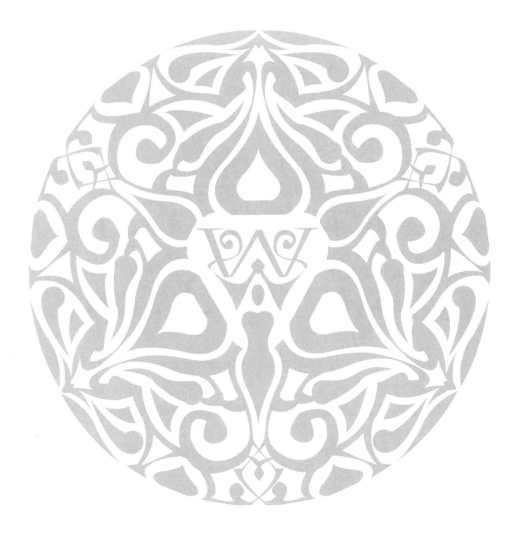

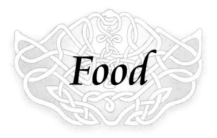

Food

Take time to feel what is most natural and easy.

BETTINA VITELL
A Taste of Heaven and Earth[1]

RESTORING PELVIC ORGAN SUPPORT requires that we *enliven* our entire digestive tract. This is because a distended, sagging stomach presses on our bowels, which in turn press against our pelvic organs. We can't expect to change the condition of our pelvic organs unless we're prepared to tone our gut as well. Just like our buttocks or biceps, our stomach and bowels are capable of shaping up, becoming firmer and more resilient.

Lively food is whole, natural, organic, locally grown, in season, nutrient-packed, and enzyme-rich. This food will provide the vital forces necessary to strengthen tissues, normalize cells, and energize organs, bringing the pelvic floor back toward a state of primal health.

Just as there are a multitude of cultures in the world, so are there a myriad of natural diets that heal and nourish the human body. Americans have a problem with "natural food," however, as George Ohsawa pointed out several decades ago: "The strangest thing in the West, it would appear to me, is the total absence of the most fundamental concept of living, namely principal food. My most significant discovery in America, fully as important as the one made by Christopher Columbus, is that here the idea of principle food has completely disappeared. No professor or man of medicine nowadays seems to be aware of its great value."[2]

Americans may be a bit confused about what constitutes healthful food, yet never before in history have we had the information, experience, and validation to help us understand and choose a healing, restorative diet. Twenty years ago it was common for someone interested in health food to become either a raw-foodist, macrobiotic, or vegan. We now know there is value in all these paths and can learn from the lives and deaths of those who follow them.

The German healer Arnold Ehret followed a strictly raw food diet composed primarily of fruit. He claimed to have tremendous health and energy, yet died at age fifty-six of a fractured skull after falling off a curb while walking. Fruit is very deficient in calcium, and unless combined with green leafy vegetables, will place the body in negative calcium balance. It is doubtful such a fall would have been fatal if Ehret's bones were strong and healthy.

George Ohsawa, founder of macrobiotics, proposed a traditional Japanese diet of brown rice, fermented soy foods, seafoods, cooked vegetables, and green tea. This diet worked well for him throughout his life, keeping him free from common ailments and allowing him great energy for his work, although he died at age seventy-two of a massive cardiovascular event. We now know vitamin C and associated bioflavonoids, best supplied by raw plant food and largely destroyed by cooking, are the substances that keep the connective tissue of our blood vessels strong and supple.

Traditional vegetarian diets that rely heavily on cooked grains, legumes, heated oils, boiled milk, and cooked vegetables are often devoid of enzymes, substances made only by living organisms and contained only in raw food. Enzymes initiate all life processes, including the digestion of food. Raw food contains the very enzymes our bodies need to digest it. Cooked, pasteurized, and processed foods no longer contain their original enzyme content, so the pancreas must work hard to produce a steady supply of digestive enzymes as the liver struggles to detoxify altered fats and proteins. Pancreatic and liver cancers are common in cultures that rely heavily on cooked food.

Nathan Pritikin, famous for his grain-based, low-fat, low-protein, vegan diet cured himself of heart disease, but died in his sixties of leukemia. Grains are great for birds that possess a unique organ (a *crop*) for sprouting them before they are digested, but pose a special problem for humans. Their outer layers (bran) contain enzyme inhibitors that keep the seed from sprouting under the wrong conditions. Although this fiber can help us in some ways, it can also cause severe intestinal irritation. The gluten, or protein portion of grain, is a common allergen for many people causing bloating, cramping, and diarrhea. Grains also contain phytates, substances that bind with many minerals in the gut and carry them out of our body. Unless properly prepared and eaten with discretion, grains can weaken the digestive system and compromise immunity.

The healthiest and longest living among us appear to be those who eat a high proportion of raw plant food with an emphasis on leafy greens, fruit, oils in their original form (whole, raw nuts, seeds, avocados, coconuts), and young shoots and seedlings (sprouts). We have recent examples of raw foodists who lived very long lives and died while still actively engaged in living. Norman Walker, health activist, author, and inventor of the Norwalk juicing machine, died sharp and alert while working at his desk at age one hundred nine. Raw juice and salads had comprised his entire diet for almost three-quarters of a century.

If we consider the fossil record, it is well understood that our earliest ancestors ate diets composed of fruit, green leaves, and insects.[3] Insects provided the human diet extra calcium and magnesium, as well as plentiful amounts of vitamin B$_{12}$, the substance that protects the myelin sheath surrounding our nerve cells. The only vitamin known to contain its own mineral co-factor (cobalt), B$_{12}$, is synthesized inside bacteria that live in the digestive systems of insects and animals. Vitamin B$_{12}$ is plentiful in unwashed fruits and vegetables, and naturally stored, unfumigated grain.

Humans have been eating meat successfully for perhaps 100,000 years. Charred animal flesh, however, is just as toxic to our intestinal tract today as it always has been. Early cultures dried most of the meat and fish they didn't eat raw; they learned to cook grains and beans. Thousands of varieties of wild plants composed the major part of prehistoric diets, and it is estimated that in North America alone between 3,000 and 5,000 wild plants were probably used as food by indigenous peoples.[4]

Dairy products were incorporated into our diets much later, about 10,000 to 15,000 years ago. Only a few cultures utilized animal milk, developing the enzyme lactase to digest it. The majority of people worldwide continue to have a severe intolerance to milk sugar.

When people lived in small groups, all members of the band or tribe had a similar physique and constitution and everyone within the group ate the same food. As groups began to travel, exchange members, and absorb one another, different constitutions and tolerances became co-existent within the same communities. As agriculture gained a strong foothold, populations grew very large, and people were subject to a greater threat from disease-producing microorganisms than they had been while in small, mobile groups. People learned that if they boiled their water and cooked all their food, many of the sicknesses they were familiar with could be prevented. Thus, the earliest and most natural human diets gave way to the safe, storable, portable, creative, and stimulating food of civilization.

After years of experimenting with my own diet, I've found a balance between raw and cooked food that keeps me feeling vital and energized. I eat a raw breakfast (usually figs, almonds, apples in winter, or cantaloupe in summer), raw lunch (pumpkin seeds, sun dried tomatoes, dulse, avocado), and a mostly cooked dinner (raw or steamed greens, ground seeds, sea vegetables, beans, and grains). Understanding the futility of trying to prescribe a single diet for everyone, Udo Erasmus put it best: "Natural diets of traditional people living in different areas indicate that human digestion is versatile, and adapts to subsist on foods that grow in the location, climate, and environment to which (our food) plants and animals became adapted."[5] Each of us must choose our own diet depending on preferences, tolerances, abilities, and resources. Give yourself freedom to find your own metabolic balance, as only you know what keeps you feeling well.

We live at a time of easy access to information about traditional food systems as well as research from the fields of biochemistry and nutritional science. Not since we were one with our original diets have so many people been better able to fulfill our bodies' nutritional needs,† which include:

---

† *I am well aware of the many people among us who do not have the resources to locate and afford quality food.*

- Twenty-one minerals
- Thirteen vitamins
- Eight amino acids
- Two fatty acids
- A clean-burning source of fuel (carbohydrate)
- Water
- Oxygen
- Light[6]

Because our natural environment has been greatly altered, we may now benefit from foods and substances we probably didn't require only a few generations ago:

- Mineral supplements
- Radioprotective foods

And we are wise to avoid foods that may harbor damaging agents:

- Animal fat
- Imported food
- Genetically modified organisms

Minerals

The major minerals needed by humans are calcium, magnesium, nitrogen, phosphorus, potassium, and sulfur. Trace elements necessary for health and longevity include iron, zinc, copper, manganese, boron, molybdenum, chlorine, sodium, cobalt, silicon, iodine, selenium, chromium, nickel, and arsenic. To say we need "minerals" might give rise to the impression that we can satisfy our body's requirement for them by simply swallowing elemental mineral supplements or by eating mineral-fortified food.

This is not the case, however, since the minerals our bodies require are biologically combined with enzymes through the work of microorganisms in soil. It is only minerals in this organic form (mettalo-enzymes) that orchestrate life processes, including metabolism; cardiovascular, nerve, and immune function; cell production; and detoxification.[7] Enzymes made by our bodies also need a mineral "co-factor" to carry out their functions successfully. Over eighty human enzymes are known to require zinc to function properly, while many others utilize magnesium and copper.[8] To stay healthy, most of our minerals must come from the food we eat.

Vitamins

In the same way minerals cannot be utilized in their elemental form, vitamins cannot be used by our body in pure crystalline form. Rather, they are attached by plant processes with phytochemicals or by bacterial processes with other micronutrients in an intricate "complex" that is impossible to duplicate in a laboratory.[9] We have learned that vitamin and mineral deficiencies are not curable by giving single nutrient replacement (only the deficient vitamin or mineral), but that several additional elements are also required to correct a single deficiency.

Most vitamins are heat sensitive, particularly vitamins C, B_6, and folic acid, which are destroyed by cooking. Not only should our vitamins come from food, but that food should be as fresh and unaltered as possible. Most people in the industrialized world die of degenerative diseases caused by chronic deficiencies in essential nutrients. A diet rich in whole, unprocessed, lively food assures that our bodies receive what nature intended.

Amino Acids

Most of the world lives well on far less protein than the average American. Our cultural hypnosis has us believing in the "protein myth" established during the latter half of the twentieth century by the National Egg Board, the National Dairy Council, and the National Livestock and Meat Board.[10]

The truth is that we only need about thirty grams of protein a day (about the weight of ten pennies) to maintain excellent health, which is best provided by plant food. The eight essential amino acids are found in a wide variety of plants and are easily supplied by a wholesome, varied diet. In other words, it is not necessary to worry about a protein deficiency unless one is on the brink of starvation.

The high protein diets of the West contribute to the development of osteoporosis by increasing the acidity of our blood. Our bodies respond by drawing alkaline calcium from our bones in order to re-establish normal pH. For decades women have been told to drink a quart of milk a day to increase bone density, when in fact protein-rich cow's milk worsens negative calcium balance and heightens the risk for osteoporosis.[11]

Fatty Acids

We are beginning to understand that our civilization's craving for protein is actually a craving for fat, and our people, engorged in calories, are actually fat-starved. This is because *quality* sources of the two essential fats our bodies do not manufacture, and therefore must come from food, are in short supply in the modern Western diet. These are Omega-6† fatty acid found in many seeds, including sunflower, pumpkin, corn, and sesame, and Omega-3 fatty acid, contained in fish, hemp seed, flax seed, chia seed, wal-

---

† *The standard American diet actually contains excessive amounts of altered Omega-6 fatty acid in the form of bottled safflower, corn, sunflower, soybean, and cottonseed oils. These oils pose a health risk, especially when heated.*

nuts, wheat germ, and green leafy vegetables. Omega-3 used to be abundant in early diets as coastal people traded fish, inland people traded flax and hemp seed, and all ate large amounts of succulent green herbs. The role these fats play within our bodies cannot be overstated as they assist in carrying out the most vital of life processes, including energy production, oxygen transfer, red blood cell production, growth, cell division, sexual function, and brain development.[12]

Like vitamins, essential fatty acids (EFAs) are destroyed by heat, light, and oxygen, and should be consumed in the most unaltered way possible. Most bottled vegetable oils have been subjected to a whole range of de-naturing processes and are unfit for human consumption. Hydrogenated fats (margarines and shortenings) are made by changing the molecular structure of plant oils into substances that do not occur in nature. These clog and confuse our metabolic pathways, leading to many degenerative conditions including cancer and cardiovascular disease.[13]

High-quality, cold pressed olive oil is healthful to consume in moderation, but is not an essential fat (our body can construct monounsaturated fat from its own raw material), and excessive amounts can cause imbalances in the natural processes carried out by EFAs.

Fuel

Glucose, the basic energy unit of the body, is best supplied by a diet rich in fruit and complex carbohydrates. Complex carbohydrates such as brown rice, millet, barley, and wheat, when combined with quality vegetable protein and essential fat, are digested slowly, producing even energy states and mood.

There was a time before agriculture when we ate far less grains and beans than we do today, and it is beneficial to understand how best to utilize these now important foods. Grains are kind of a mixed blessing. Highly economical, convenient, delicious, and nutritious, they can also cause difficulty if not prepared and eaten with discretion. Grains contain phytates, substances known to carry minerals (zinc, iron, magnesium) out of our bodies. Phytic acid is such a strong magnetizer of minerals that it is used in the oil industry to clear vegetable oil of its cloudy mineral content. Phytates can be neutralized by soaking whole grain or flour overnight in water, and then proceeding with further preparation. The protein portion (gluten) of grains is an allergen for many people. We usually develop allergies to substances our immune system is overwhelmed with, and wheat is one of the worst offenders. Wheat is on American tables at every meal as bread, cereal, crackers, cookies, gravies, soups, stews, batters, and desserts. Limiting and rotating consumption of grains helps increase our tolerance to them.

Beans contain enzyme inhibitors that are only deactivated by soaking; therefore, all beans should be soaked overnight before cooking. The soaking water should be discarded and the beans covered with fresh water for cooking. Adding a handful of dried seaweed to the cooking water (I prefer kombu) provides trace minerals, deactivates the gas-forming quality of beans, and deepens their flavor.

Water, Oxygen & Light

One rarely thinks of food as a source of water, oxygen, and light, yet food is actually one of the greatest sources of these life-giving factors. In nature, animals only drink when thirsty, the greater proportion of their water needs met by the food they consume. Mountain gorillas, which subsist primarily on fruit, quench their thirst by dipping their hand in a stream of water and then licking the droplets off the back of their hairy hand. If we take our cues from nature, it may well be unhealthful to guzzle water from plastic bottles throughout the day, forcing large amounts of fluid through the fine meshwork of our kidneys. The water contained in fruits and vegetables is pure and plentiful.

Green leaves and fresh fruit are some of the best ways we can increase the amount of clean oxygen into our system. Pure oxygen molecules are incorporated into the matrix of the plant itself and released when we eat the food. One of the biggest changes I noticed when I increased the amount of raw green plant food in my diet was that I began to breathe more deeply. I never again questioned the oxygen-carrying capacity of plant food.

Every type of food we eat, whether fresh, dewy kale leaves from the garden, or hamburgers from fast-food restaurant chains, is transformed light energy from the sun. The only difference is how light or dark that energy is. When we eat low on the food chain or close to the source of our energy, there is a vital quality to our food that is progressively diminished as it is cycled through animals and industry.

Pure light energy from the sun comes to us in full spectrum color and is utilized by each energy center of our body. Our adrenal glands, the largest users of vitamin C, benefit from a diet rich in red fruits (apples, cherries, berries, rose hips.) Our uterus and ovaries require large amounts of vitamin A, richly supplied by orange fruits and vegetables (apricots, yams, carrots, squash.) Our pancreas, which orchestrates digestion, thrives on the energy of yellow grains and golden seed oils. Our heart and thymus must have abundant calcium and magnesium to function, best supplied by dark, leafy greens. The blues and violets used by our higher energy centers abound in iodine-rich seaweeds, cabbages, kales, and hibiscus. If color were our only guide to a healthful and balanced diet, which it probably was long ago, we would undoubtedly fare very well.

Mineral Supplements

Supplementing our diets with high-quality, biocompatible (chelated) minerals has become increasingly important for three reasons. First, our nation's farmland has long been exhausted of its original mineral content. Minerals are not replaced as they used to be through natural composting methods, so our soil remains deficient in both major and trace minerals. Modern agriculture replaces only three minerals—nitrogen, phosphorus, and potassium—through chemical fertilizers. Secondly, modern hybrid varieties of grains and vegetables have been developed for big yields by increasing their carbohydrate content, while lowering their mineral content. Lastly, force-feeding of petrol-based fertilizers causes plants to be filled up with nitrogenous substances instead of a wide variety of essential nutrients.[14]

Although it is important to try to obtain the greater part of our mineral requirement from the food we eat, it may also be necessary to treat such symptoms as heart palpitations (magnesium/calcium), thyroid dysfunction (iodine), poor wound healing (zinc), and fatigue (iron), with dietary supplements.

Radioprotective Food

We have always been exposed to certain levels of natural or background radiation from both the earth itself and the cosmos. Man-made radiation has increased drastically however, and the levels of radioactive substances we are now subject to are far greater than ever before in our evolution.

First-hand experience with survivors of Hiroshima and Nagasaki, as well as research into radioprotective substances, have given us an awareness of foods that both prevent radioactive minerals from entering our tissues and carry these same "hot" minerals out of our bodies.

If we do not maintain a steady supply of stable elements such as calcium, iodine, and iron in our diets, chances are increased that our bodies will take up and try to utilize their radioactive counterparts—strontium-90, iodine-131, and plutonium—which now are ubiquitous in our environment. Many substances found in whole, natural foods are known to remove radioactive elements from our intestinal tract. A diet rich in grains, beans, fresh fruit (especially apples), vegetables (especially cabbage), seeds, nuts, seaweed, and miso (a fermented soy food) will help minimize our environmental exposure to ionizing radiation.[15]

Animal Fat

There was a time when animal fat contributed to human health and longevity. Long ago when people ate meat raw or dried, the qualities of animal fat were pure, unaltered, and utilized for energy as well as many other life processes. Today, by every measure, most animal fat poses serious risk to health. From the way it is raised to the way it is prepared, animal fat is altered at the molecular level and is a potential source of an array of toxic and destructive chemicals.

Petroestrogens (sometimes called xenoestrogens) may be some of the most damaging substances contained in animal fat. Products of the burgeoning plastics and pesticide industries, petroestrogens move around the planet undeterred and are stored most notably in the fat tissue and mammary secretions of animals. These hormone-disrupting chemicals are thought to play a significant role in women's diseases including breast cancer, endometrial cancer, ovarian cancer, menstrual irregularities, thyroid disturbances, and miscarriage.[16]

Imported Food

A generation ago we gave little thought to where our food was grown. That it arrived at our grocery store fresh, tasty, and attractive was all that really mattered. As with many other aspects of modern life, our food sources have been affected by overcrowding, poor sanitation, and chemical pollution.

Fresh fruits and vegetables have now joined meat, eggs, and dairy products as potential harbingers of dangerous pathogens. Outbreaks of salmonella have been traced to tomatoes, mustard greens, bean sprouts, cantaloupe, and watermelon. Shigella has been linked to onions. Cabbage and lettuce have been found to contain listeriosis, and hepatitis A has occasionally contaminated green onions and strawberries.[17] The benefits of buying food locally often include cost savings, higher vitamin and mineral content, and less chance of serious contamination with disease-causing microorganisms, pesticide residue, and toxic sludge.

Genetically Modified Organisms

The last decades of the twentieth century witnessed funding of several large bioengineering firms to develop changes to the gene structure of many of our basic food plants. Using the same restrictive, abstract science that has brought us single-species forestry, hydroelectric dams on all our major rivers, and nuclear waste, the genetic engineers are carrying out their mission quite "successfully."

Their most widely propagated experiment, carried out on corn, envisions vast stretches of herbicide-resistant fields that remain unaffected when heavily sprayed with glyphosphate weed killers. Instead of moving farmers away from dependence on chemical pesticides, modified crops encourage pesticide use, further threatening the world's water supply, food supply, and wildlife.

Second in acreage only to herbicide-resistant crops, plants are now engineered to produce toxin in their own tissues, including the parts of the plant used for food by humans. *Bacillus thuringiensis* (Bt), a bacterium that naturally produces toxin when activated by the gastric juices of certain insects, has been genetically integrated into the tissues of corn, canola, potatoes, and cotton, making these plants poisonous to the insects that feed on them. In contrast to Bt spray, which organic farmers have been selectively employing for decades, genetically engineered plants produce fully active toxin that does not require activation by the digestive systems of insects. Recent studies from Cornell University and

Iowa State University have confirmed that the pollen from Bt corn can kill Monarch butterflies.[18] Bt toxin also leeches into the soil from plant roots, possibly harming soil microorganisms.[19]

Because genetic engineering is imprecise and unpredictable, little is known of additional risks to human health the altered plants may pose. Corn is a wind-pollinated crop, and it has already proven impossible to keep organic and unmodified varieties uncontaminated by gene-spliced ones. This will be true for many other plants that join the Next Great Experiment, the most onerous risk being new, unproven varieties of food and fiber plants eventually replacing the natural gene pool of their wild and traditionally cultivated relatives.

Each year in late summer, I drive the back roads of New Mexico to Señor Sena's farm on the Pecos River. Along with pinto beans, several types of native chili, and Señora Sena's spectacular sunflower-sized marigolds, the old farmer grows an heirloom variety of white corn that his father, and his father before that, grew on the same breathtaking piece of land. Señor lets the long, slender ears of corn dry on the stalk, harvests them by hand, and after mechanically removing the seeds from the cob, fills dozens of burlap sacks to sell.

I grind the corn in my electric "stone" mill throughout the winter, turning it into mouthwatering polenta, tamales, breads, and cakes. The taste, texture, and aroma of the corn transcends words, and the thought of ever eating regular yellow field corn again is unbearable. Señor's two daughters live and work in Albuquerque at computer-related jobs. Neither has any interest in taking over the family farm, which will one day quietly recede back into the banks of the Pecos as so many have before it. Always careful to save a few seeds each spring to plant on my rocky hilltop, I know full well the impossibility of sustaining the bounty, the lusciousness, and the awesome complexity of my Pecos River Valley corn as grown by Señor Sena.

Food is sacred. Our most tangible link with the divine, every mouthful we take is a communion between creator and creation. Coming back to a place of health means first reconnecting with our food. It is precisely this relationship that will bring our bodies back toward the natural design intended by our evolution.

❧

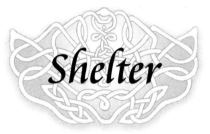

Shelter

Everywhere in these days men have, in their mockery, ceased to understand that the true security is to be found in social solidarity rather than in isolated individual effort. But this terrible individualism must inevitably have an end, and all will suddenly understand how unnaturally they are separated from one another. It will be the spirit of the time, and people will marvel that they have sat so long in darkness without seeing the light.

F. M. Dostoevsky
The Brothers Karamazov[1]

WE NOW KNOW THAT PROBLEMS with pelvic organ support arise from medical interventions and lifestyle habits. As we work toward correcting habitual patterns within our own bodies, we must also look around us for further ways to support total well-being. Encompassed by vast material wealth, unparalleled convenience, and "insurance" against any of it ever changing, our "privileged" society is far less supported by our surroundings than ever before in human existence. In terms of true safety and security, most of us are absolutely impoverished. Consider the whole concept of shelter or "the state of being covered or protected."† Although we've been "educated" to believe that early cultures lived lives filled with hardship and brutality, several investigators refute this notion.[2] Tribal communities worldwide have always provided, and many continue to provide, cradle-to-grave support and connection for their members. Profound knowledge of the natural world gives them a level of security relatively unknown in modern society. Spiritual connection and a deep reverence for life have sustained them since the dawn of humanity. I remember how astonished I was to read Jack Kornfield's account of just how sheltered a human being can be, as he described a tribe in east Africa where:

> *The birth date of a child is not counted from the day of its physical birth nor even the day of conception, as in other village cultures. For this tribe the birth date comes the first time the child is a thought in its mother's mind. Aware of her intention to conceive a child with a particular father, the mother then goes off to*

sit alone under a tree. There she sits and listens until she can hear the song of the child that she hopes to conceive. Once she has heard it, she returns to her village and teaches it to the father so that they can sing it together as they make love, inviting the child to join them. After the child is conceived, she sings it to the baby in her womb. Then she teaches it to the old women and midwives of the village, so that throughout the labor and at the miraculous moment of birth itself, the child is greeted with its song. After the birth all the villagers learn the song of their new member and sing it to the child when it falls or hurts itself. It is sung in times of triumph, or in rituals and initiations. This song becomes a part of the marriage ceremony when the child is grown, and at the end of life, his or her loved ones will gather around the deathbed and sing this song for the last time.[3]

For us, the true experience of "home" is a hazy mythology. Most of us have traveled far from our place of birth, moving several times during the course of our lives. Our parents may be living out the last years of their lives in nursing homes, and our children away at expensive colleges. We seldom have much connection with our neighbors and even less with our churches or local governments. Many of us live as captives within convenient, efficient, and totally artificial environments. We go to sleep at night on polyurethane foam mattresses between polyester-blend sheets and blankets. Artificial light and unnatural electromagnetic fields course through our brains and bodies as we breathe toxic vapors from the paints and plastics that fill our homes.

We step out of bed in the morning onto wall-to-wall carpet permeated with formaldehyde that outgases over many years. Breakfast consists of de-natured foods from boxes, cans, and plastic containers. We clean our homes with disinfectants, detergents, and polishes containing extremely dangerous chemicals like benzene, toluene, and dioxin. Although well-known to be carcinogenic (cancer-causing), mutagenic (DNA destroying), and teratogenic (birth defect-producing), habit and convenience blind us to the health risks these products pose.

We drive our car about town and in one year release its own weight in carbon into the atmosphere, our personal contribution to global warming.[4] Our manicured lawns and gardens are often sprayed with toxic pesticides and fungicides. We cook our food in microwave ovens, destroying its natural life-giving qualities and possibly exposing ourselves to dangerous radiation. We then store the leftovers in soft plastics, permeated with hormone-disrupting chemicals.

Does any of this matter? Are we really affected by living in such a synthetic world? Voices from every corner of the planet have begun to echo a resounding YES to both these questions. Not only have there been tremendous increases in cancers and birth defects in recent decades, but our mental health resembles that of captive wild animals whose behaviors have been carefully observed in zoos for over a century. Cindy Engel in her book *Wild Health,* tells us that almost 10 percent of Americans have a classifiable anxiety disorder and "With our neuroses, self-abuse, eating disorders, addictions, and depression, humans look frighteningly like captive wild animals prevented from invoking their natural coping strategies."[5]

Disconnected from a universal, abiding perspective, hypnotized and poisoned by our contraptions and consumptions, we've become active participants in what has become known as the "culture of violence." E.F. Schumacher told us in the 1970s that "The system of nature, of which man is a part, tends to be self-balancing, self-adjusting, self-cleaning. Not so with technology... Technology recognizes no self-limiting principle—in terms, for instance, of size, speed, or violence... Technology, and in particular the super-technology of the modern world, acts like a foreign body, and there are now numerous signs of rejection.[6]

A generation later, Chellis Glendinning relates how we're doing in our brave, new world:

> Previously an injured or nightmare-ridden person might visit a medicine woman once or twice, enter into a ceremony for a moon, or take an infusion of plant medicine. But now the experience of trauma was becoming all too commonplace—until today when we live almost entirely apart from natural rhythms, encased almost entirely in technological environments and mechanistic social forms, subject to an entire system caught in a seemingly unending cycle of abuse. As the aftershocks of our collective trauma have become 'normal' fare for our psyches, healing ourselves has become a life-long task.[7]

If domestication is the cause of so much ill health, what would it take to become less captive, freer, wilder, more natural? David Suzuki and Peter Knudtson ventured to answer that question in their book *Wisdom of the Elders*. They identified a "native mind," or way of seeing reality, shared by traditional peoples the world over. This perspective includes a deep reverence for nature, a sense that spirit is dispersed throughout the cosmos, and the notion that there is great wisdom in the natural world and in natural processes. Time is seen as circular, and humans bestowed with responsibility to care for themselves, each other, the planet, and future generations. The Yarrelin people of Northern Australia express this idea poignantly: "All that preceded us and all that comes after depends on us. What we do matters so powerfully that to evade our responsibilities is to call down chaos."[8]

Our own health and the health of the planet is gravely threatened by the massive ways in which we've manipulated nature. Our connections with the earth, natural processes, and our own bodies are lost, forgotten, and relegated to "experts." To become well we must connect with our body and our home. Early peoples deeply comprehended their homeland from the soil and water under their feet to the air and stars overhead. They understood that all of nature is alive and animated by a single unifying force and that all health influenced by subtle energies in both positive and negative ways.

In his groundbreaking work *Vibrational Medicine*, Richard Gerber describes how the molecular arrangement of the physical body is actually a complex network of interwoven energy fields. Subtle vibrational energies flowing down from the cosmos, rising up from deep in the earth, and contained within natural food, coordinate electrophysiologic and hormonal functions and organize cellular structures within the physical body. It's from a disturbance at these subtle levels that illness originates.[9] Tuning into life's subtle, yet vital energies is something we can begin to do right now wherever we are. It's as easy as stopping to listen to the rhythm of our own breath, sitting still outside under a full moon, or trying to feel love actually flowing out from our heart.

In order to support the subtle energies that carry essential, healing information, our environment needs to be cleared of the congestive, polluting energies of technology. The best way to begin to bring about this change is to create a sanctuary in the room where we spend most of our lives—the bedroom. Our own bioelectric system (alpha and beta waves) vibrates at the same rate as the earth's electromagnetic field. When we sleep with our head to the north, we align our energies with the natural pulse of the planet. When we reduce electromagnetic "smog" by eliminating TVs, electric heaters, electric blankets, and electric clocks from the bedroom, we also alleviate a significant amount of biological stress.[10] Peace, clarity, and vitality are our natural birthright, not merely the occasional experience of wilderness.

It is vitally important to reduce exposure to artificial light as much as possible when we sleep. The *Journal of the National Cancer Institute* revealed a recent study, concluding that women who are exposed to artificial light at night are at greater risk of developing breast cancer.[11] Ancient Vedic tradition teaches that the pineal gland is awake even when our eyes are closed and we are asleep. Seasonal changes and perhaps a wealth of other information is picked up by the pineal from the light of the moon and the stars. It is possible that our very evolution is inextricably woven with the movements, events, and processes of the celestial bodies. It is best to have no light pollution inside or outside our room, and to sleep with windows open to the night sky. If this is not possible, total darkness will suffice until healthier changes can be made. It is also important to expose as much skin as possible to the sun for at least a few minutes each day, stimulating the pineal to release the sleep-inducing hormone, melatonin, at night.

Remove all books from the bedroom and anything else that collects dust. Make sure your bedding is made from natural fibers and always wash them in natural soap without perfumes, bleach, softeners, etc. Floors can be compressed earth, wood, clay tile, or carpet covered with cotton throw rugs to keep from breathing synthetic fibers. When you sleep on your side, place a pillow under your head and one between your knees. This keeps the accessory muscles of your hips and buttocks aligned and unstressed, further increasing the healing capacity of the pelvic floor. Try not to use a pillow when sleeping on your back. If we elevate our head on a pillow while on our back both the natural thoracic curve and lumbar curve in our spine are strained, directing unhealthy forces to the pelvic floor.

We can clean our houses with baking soda, white vinegar, liquid soap (a plant-based soap, not a petroleum-based detergent), lemon juice, saltwater, hydrogen peroxide, pumice stone, boiling water, borax, linseed oil, and beeswax. These disinfect, degrease, demineralize, shine, and polish without harm to surfaces, groundwater, or us. Our grandmothers and their grandmothers used these products to clean and beautify their homes without the dangers and discomforts of harsh chemicals. We've become maladapted to unnatural cleaning substances and think it's normal to cough, sniffle, and sneeze while cleaning. The following list of natural cleaners will leave your house clean, your immune system unharmed, and your nervous system unstressed.

- *Baking soda* is a deodorizer and mild abrasive that absorbs odors and cleans sinks, tubs, toilets, and faucets. It's very inexpensive. Look for the economy-size box at discount stores and co-ops.

- *Distilled white vinegar* is mildly acidic and can be used full strength on chrome, porcelain, and tile for dissolving mineral deposits and soap film. Mix half and half with water and a drop of soap for a terrific window cleaner.

- *Liquid castile soap* is plant-based. It's fat-soluble, which means it effectively dissolves grease and oil. This is the best everyday cleaner for dishes, clothes, floor, sink, toilet, and bathtub. Dr. Bronner's Sal Suds™ (available in natural food stores) is a good brand to look for. Other environmentally friendly cleaners are Shaklee™ products, available from local distributors. I prefer to use one high-quality soap for all my cleaning needs.

- *Lemon juice* deodorizes and removes mineral build-up, tarnish, and grease. Brass and copper can be shined by rubbing with baking soda and a lemon wedge. Make a paste of lemon juice and salt for heavy corrosion.

- *Saltwater* disinfects by destroying bacteria through dehydration. Combine one tablespoon salt and one pint water in a spray bottle for use on stove, faucets, and refrigerator.

- *Hydrogen peroxide* should be used instead of bleach to remove bloodstains on clothing or bedding (bleach is damaging to fabric and our immunity).

- *Pumice stone* is a volcanic rock obtainable at many drug stores. This works wonders for removing the ring of hard mineral deposits in toilet bowls. It's softer than porcelain and will not scratch.

- *Boiling water* can be heated in a teapot and poured into the toilet bowl each morning to help disinfect and keep it clean.

- *Borax* is a mineral mined in the desert and is a natural and effective insecticide. It kills cockroaches by destroying their digestive system after they lick the mineral off their feet. Borax is also known to be an effective disinfectant and mold remover.

- *Linseed oil* is pressed from flaxseed. Mixed with beeswax and turpentine (a solvent derived from pine trees), it is an excellent floor and furniture wax.

If you want to make this yourself, melt the beeswax (available from woodworker supply companies, some candle companies, co-ops, and craft stores) slowly on low heat in a double boiler. *NEVER WARM BEESWAX ON DIRECT HEAT.* Remove from the heat and then slowly add a bit of turpentine. The turpentine softens the wax and makes the polish easier to apply. Once the melted wax and turpentine are fully mixed, add linseed oil in the amount of about half the volume you have in wax and turpentine. Be sure to use only *raw* linseed oil as *boiled* linseed oil has been treated with heavy metals to aid drying. Let cool and test the consistency. If too stiff, melt and add more turpentine and linseed oil. If too soft, add more wax. *ALWAYS USE A DOUBLE BOILER OR WATER BATH.* Also, the rags you use with this wax can spontaneously combust if stored improperly. Therefore, never store them or throw them in the trash after use. I burn mine in a woodstove but as an alternative, keep them in a jar half full of water until ready to discard.

The collective hallucination of our culture has us convinced that our high "standard of living" gives us something the rest of the world should envy. That "something" is an easiness, which in time turns to weakness. Down through the ages of human existence, work, rest, and pleasure flowed into each other as one continuous river of life. People didn't wish working hours away, but rather took pride in the everyday cadence and products of their endeavors. That we no longer feel the real necessity to work (other than to pay for what we buy) is in a sense self-defeating. A definition of energy, the stuff of which we are made, is "the capacity to do work."† Dissociating from work disconnects us from our true human purpose.

One possible reason many Americans are unhappy, uncomfortable, and unfulfilled by their work is put forth by Wendell Berry:

> *The growth of the exploiters' revolution on this continent has been accompanied by the growth of the idea that work is beneath human dignity, particularly any form of hand work. We have made it our overriding ambition to escape work, and as a consequence have debased work until it is only fit to escape from.*[12]

Where well-wrought American shelters were once places that responded to the requirements of their natural surroundings as well as the needs of the people who inhabited them, now they are largely a response to affluence and the social status of their owners.

The deep contentment a true sense of home can still provide was eloquently written to me in a letter by my friend and college roommate who recently expressed:

> *I was talking with a friend whom I had not seen in a while and she asked me what was new. I decided that nothing was new and that was good. We're at*

---

† *Webster's New World Dictionary*

the "move through school, animals, chores" stage and new is usually trouble. You know, like, "Oh, we're digging a new set of leach lines," or "The goats just figured a new way out of the pen." This part of our lives is centered around equipping the boys to be God honoring young men, equipped to stand tall and true. I love doing this. I know 'new' will come and I will then do things differently, but for now I am so content to be in God's will here at home.

Here in the Southwest, traditional peoples of this land taught their women to be strong and able workers. Kimberly Buchanan shares with us, "Even though domestic chores were stressed, maturing Apache girls were encouraged to develop their physical strength. They received the same basic training as boys, and all learned to be strong and vigorous. The girls were told to 'rise early, run often, and shun no hard work.'"[13] Among the pueblo cultures of the Rio Grande River Valley, it is the women who repair and maintain the earthen shelters commonly referred to as "adobes." Becky Bee, author and founder of an organization dedicated to building hand-made earthen houses for and with women tells us, "Throughout history, women have worked together homemaking, farming, cooking, and raising children. This is the glue of community. Today in the modern western world, most women are isolated from one another and are usually dependent on men and/ or the patriarchal system for their shelter."[14]

As women healing from medical violence, and as a country struggling to maintain equilibrium within a world hungry for justice, never has our need for true shelter been greater. Only by the rules of natural law can shelter be perpetually maintained. Stuart Kauffman, one of the most brilliant scientists of our time muses:

"Friend, you cannot even predict the motions of three coupled pendula. You have hardly a prayer with three mutually gravitating objects. We let loose pesticides on our crops; the insects become ill and are eaten by birds that sicken and die, allowing the insects to proliferate in increased abundance. The crops are destroyed. So much for control. Bacon, you were brilliant, but the world is more complex than your philosophy."[15]

℘

Build A Sandy Creek Bed

Several years ago I had a truckload of sand delivered to my yard, raked it into a long stretch, and planted wild flowers along either side. On sunny days I walk barefoot and relaxed up and down my "creek bed," slowly soaking up healing earth energies through the warm, soothing sand.

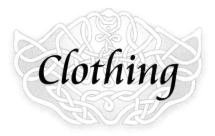

Clothing

Our clothing is a self-created environment over which we have total control.

ANITA LUVERA MAYER
Clothing From the Hands That Weave[1]

AFTER STRUGGLING WITH MY PROLAPSE for several years the day finally arrived when I realized I could no longer tolerate any constriction whatsoever around my torso. I came to this conclusion after watching the powerful impact clothes had on my condition. Tight jeans and waisted pants were immediately obvious problems, as they literally squeezed my uterus out of my body. It took longer to come to terms with the fact that anything around my waist—even stretchy tights—had a similar effect if worn for several hours. Consequently, waist-high underwear, tights, pantyhose, pants, and waist-dependent skirts were no longer viable clothing options for me.

I'm eternally grateful for having learned to sew when I was a young mother. The first garment I ever made was a maternity dress and those same skills I use today to sew almost all my own clothing. I can't imagine not being able to buy beautiful fabric for a specific style I have in mind and then use quiet evening hours to put together a dress or pair of pants that fit just right.

I've learned that stabilizing pelvic organ support is synonymous with returning to all that is natural, including the clothing we wear on our bodies. Synthetic fabrics may have looked like an ideal solution for the post-WWII woman who was reaching for ever-increasing convenience, timesaving strategies, and efficiency. The chemical industry obliged by offering her a whole array of cheap, abundant thermoplastics derived from petrochemicals. Nylon, polyester, and acrylic may look novel, glamorous, and sometimes even feel like natural fiber, but in actuality they are hazardous and polluting to both humans and the environment.

Containing polyvinyl chloride (PVC), formaldehyde, and acrylonitrile, these fabrics continuously give off vapors as they warm against our skin. Tiredness, headaches, respiratory problems, and watery eyes are just some of the symptoms associated with synthetic fabrics. PVC releases vinyl chloride, which is known to cause cancer, birth defects, genetic mutation, skin diseases, and liver dysfunction. Formalin resin made from formaldehyde, a colorless, pungent gas and known carcinogen, is combined with polyester fiber in such a way that it cannot be washed out but remains for the life of the fabric.[2,3] "Permanent Press," "No Iron," and "Shrink Proof" fabrics are a result of this process.

Natural fabrics come from many different renewable resources and offer far more comfort, ease, and health than synthetics ever could. What fabric could be more soothing and pleasant against our skin than natural cotton? Although cotton is one of the most heavily sprayed agricultural products, and the environmental impact of the cotton industry significant, pesticides do wash out of its fibers, making it generally a safer choice. Cotton may be "Sanforized," a harmless process of pre-shrinking, or "Mercerized" with a non-toxic lye solution to strengthen the fabric. The organic movement is alive and well in the cotton industry as more and more farmers choose ecologically sound ways to raise their crops (see Resources).

One of the most ancient products of cultivation, linen, is produced from the inner bark of the flax plant. The thick stems are cut down and left in the field where natural bacterial action begins to separate the fibers within. The stems are then crushed, and the fibers removed, dried, spun into thread, and woven into fabric. Linen can be either beautifully draped or sharply tailored.

What we call wool is a year's growth of fiber shorn from more than two hundred breeds of sheep, longhaired goats, angora rabbits, camels, alpacas, or llamas. Wool is extremely warm, yet allows our skin to breathe and to wick moisture. It also retains its insulating ability when wet. Raw wool containing dirt, leaves, twigs, burrs, etc., is washed in an alkaline solution to remove these impurities. It is combed until all the fibers lay in the same direction, spun into yarn, and then woven into sturdy fabric. No synthetic fleece can compare with the warmth, comfort, and richness of wool.

Hemp is produced from the stem of the *Cannabis sativa* plant. Illegal to grow in the United States, hemp fabric is imported from around the world. I bought a bolt of organic hemp material several years ago and have sewn a variety of things from shower curtains to an elegant summer dress. Exceedingly durable and comfortable, I expect the availability of hemp to increase with time.

Silk, another ancient fabric, is cultivated from the cocoon of the silkworm caterpillar. Although silk looks delicate and fragile, this fiber is strong and washable. Ramie, also from the Far East, is hand-cultivated from a species of nettle plant indigenous to China. Both of these natural, luxurious fabrics are a worthwhile indulgence.

Humans are attracted to beautiful fabrics like we are drawn to sculpted clay, shells, flowers, and polished stones. From earliest times our clothing has provided much more than warmth and modesty. Dress is our most basic form of artistic self-expression and the primary means by which we communicate who we are, what we value, and how we relate to the world.

A natural outcome of the postural work is reconceptualizing our clothing to better support the shape of our spine and pelvis. Before the dawn of reconstructive pelvic surgery it was common for medical doctors to advise women of the important role clothing plays in the treatment of prolapse. In 1882 David Wark, M.D., wrote:

The successful treatment of severe chronic cases [of prolapse] requires more prolonged and comprehensive measures. In these cases the clothing should be supported from the shoulders by some suitable device: no pressure being permitted on the hips or abdomen.[4]

Loose-fitting dresses, jumpers and overalls fulfill Dr Wark's clothing prescription, but today's woman has a level of creative freedom unimaginable in the days of petticoats and corsets. Low-rise wrap-around skirts, tunics with leggings, and drawstring pants are just a few designs that complement the female spine and pelvis.

Whatever your clothing choices, it is important to consider the natural shape of the spine, and to dress for the comfort and mobility of our original design. Before the surgical field became the tiny window through which theories of pelvic organ support were developed during the twentieth century, earlier doctors were able to see the importance of the larger skeletal frame upon which support depends.

It is well known, but should be more constantly borne in mind, that the obliquity of the pelvis is so great that, when a women stands erect, a vertical line representing the axis of the body will, in its descent, touch the anterior surface of the 3rd lumbar vertebra, and, falling into the pelvis, will strike against the bodies of the ossa pubis [pubic bones]...The displacement of the uterus, when the organs are healthy and in a natural position, is resisted by the very weight and pressure from above, which, under other circumstances, might and often does, cause its displacement. Such are the admirable provisions made for the sustentation of the uterus. They are, indeed, so effectual that no bad effects usually result among healthy and laborious women, whether in savage or civilized life, though they are daily on their feet for many hours, and are constantly making great muscular effort in their various occupations.[5]

☙

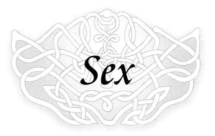

Sex

I can't forget the taste of your mouth.
From your lips
All the Heavens pour out.
I can't forget when we are one
With you alone, I am free.

CARLOS SANTANA[1]

*I*NTERFERENCE WITH SEXUAL EXPERIENCE is a common reason women opt for surgery to "correct" problems of pelvic organ support. Pelvic organ prolapse and urinary incontinence have been shrouded in secrecy for as long as Western women can remember, and promptly responded to with radical pelvic surgery. Women have no understanding of the natural history or prevalence of their disease and remain confused, embarrassed, and dependent on their doctor's advice. Scores of women then march off to the surgeon's office believing vaginoplasty will help their condition. Many return having made a true bargain with the devil.

They've traded their fully sensile, naturally contoured, completely redeemable tissues and organs for damaged nerves, disfiguring dissections, permanently irritating synthetic sutures, compromised bowel and bladder function, or perhaps complete obliteration of their sexual capacity. Where once sex was a little awkward, yet the chances of healing within reach, now it is irrevocably diminished or altogether destroyed. To quote the gynecologists once again, "Thus, when surgery is completed, what you have is what you get; the resiliency of the premenopausal resting vagina, capable of considerable stretching during coitus while still maintaining adequate support, is a luxury long gone."[2]

The overwhelming sadness with which women try to communicate the loss of their sexual function is heartbreaking. In her book *Your Guide to Hysterectomy, Ovary Removal, & Hormone Replacement*, Elizabeth Plourde expresses the pain and frustration of her own experience with hysterectomy:

> *When a woman has her uterus from the beginning of her sexuality, it is impossible to separate out, or understand, the role it plays in sexual satisfaction. Only when it is missing, can she feel the difference. The loss is tremendous. Male doctors, who are mostly*

responsible for the current philosophy that female organs are no longer necessary after childbearing years, have never felt a woman's orgasm. How can they tell women their female organs perform only one function? They cannot possibly know the feeling of an orgasm, with a uterus and cervix, nor the difference in quality without them.[3]

I find it astonishing, but not surprising, that only a handful of women have stepped forward to scream their agony at a system whereby their very womanhood is devastated. Because Western women are deeply convinced they are somehow defective, it's harder to question all the things we do to ourselves or have done to us by others to try to diminish our innate sense of shame and inadequacy for simply being who we are. I also know that it takes time to comprehend the extent of our injury. The worse that injury is, the greater our emotional devastation, and the less likely we are to fight back. I believe this dynamic has not only been recognized, but also counted on over the course of the past one hundred years of gynecologic surgery. It is of particular interest to note that Howard Kelly, one of the early founders of gynecology and creator of many of the pelvic reconstructive surgeries still in use today, is said to have been "A devout fundamentalist in religious faith, a Sunday school teacher, profoundly prudish, and deeply antisexual," and is himself quoted as saying in 1900, "I do not believe pleasure in the sexual act has any particular bearing on the happiness of life."[4]

In order to understand what happens within the pelvic area when we have sex, let's take a look at the physiology of the female sexual response cycle. In response to stimulation, if the neural pathways are undamaged, sensory signals are sent from the clitoris to the spinal cord via the pudendal nerve, and on to the brain, returning by the same route. Blood vessels that run alongside the neural pathways engorge erectile tissue in the clitoris and swell the walls of the vagina. The lower one-third of the vagina becomes full and the nerves there become very sensitive to stimulation and pressure. The clitoris and uterus begin to "talk to each other" as the round ligaments, attached to the uterus at one end and the labia at the other, begin to quicken and tug slightly back and forth. Clear fluid is forced through the vaginal walls, providing a slippery medium within. The levator ani muscles of the pelvic diaphram contract and release as excitement and stimulation continue. At the height of this accelerating muscle tension and nerve stimulation, the uterus contracts and rises out of the vagina. A series of intense rhythmic contractions are then experienced throughout the pelvic chamber and sometimes all the way to the toes.

So why would a woman ever want to give up the most pleasurable bodily sensation a human being is capable of experiencing? Yet many doctors, and indeed much of society in general, believe that as women age they voluntarily become more sexually abstinent. In one of the most important books of our time, *Passionate Marriage*, David Schnarch debunks this myth by documenting his vast experience in the field of sex therapy.[5] He assures us that sexual fulfillment is not remotely wasted on the young, but rather the best sex of our lives happens in our forties, fifties, sixties, and beyond. This is true for women as well as men. Furthermore, Schnarch elucidates how a lifelong sexually intimate relationship with one partner is really a spiritual path, providing the grist from which we transcend our own egos, and learn to truly love, trust, and give. The juxtaposition of these facts alongside the statistical reality of surgeries that compromise our capacity for sexual intimacy—more than one third of the female population by age sixty—is earthshaking. Men should be as terrified of this prospect as women.

Given that any sort of "corrective" surgery for loss of pelvic organ support is not a viable option, what are we to do about sex? We need to begin by addressing our fears. First of all, a thorough pelvic exam by a qualified women's care specialist is necessary so we can rest assured that we are sound and whole. Secondly, it is important to realize many women maintain active and satisfying sex lives while living with both prolapse and urinary incontinence. Two recent studies have shown that sexual function in women with prolapse and urinary incontinence does not differ from that in continent women without prolapse.[6,7] Understand that loss of pelvic organ support is very common among healthy women. Deepening trust and intimacy with our sexual partner by sharing openly our worries and concerns will help dismantle any barriers to a completely healthy and joyful experience. Deliberate and steady attention to diet, exercise, and posture will tone and reposition the abdominal organs as well as elevate the pelvic organs and tighten their supports. Bladder, rectum, and uterus will begin to assume their normal configuration within the pelvis. Sex is one of the best activities to aid in this process.

The myth of the too-large vagina is gaining momentum, thanks to physicians who specialize in the new trend of cosmetic vaginal surgery. Magnus Murphy, M.D., writes:

Only a male can understand (and therefore inform women) how pelvic floor sagging and a stretched vagina affect male sexual experience...something that many prolapsers or women who have had children secretly worry about. Superficial reassurances that this is not a problem is simply hogwash. This is an issue that is just as, or even more, in the closet even today. It is simply politically incorrect in many quarters to even imply such a problem exists for thousands of couples. Most males will never admit to this, knowing the pain such a statement will create. However the result may be lack of libido, a general decrease in sexual activities, or even infidelity.[8]

Thankfully, earlier doctors offered a much more realistic view on the matter: "The extent to which reconstruction of a very loose vaginal outlet will contribute to coital satisfaction has been undoubtedly overemphasized. A consensus of the more thoughtful gynecologists recognize that a noticeable looseness of the vagina is not a common cause of marital incompatibility; and as a result, prophylactic 'tightening up' of the introitus will not necessarily improve marital relations that are frayed more often by nonanatomic factors."[9]

The reason vaginal caliber does not significantly affect male sexual experience is that distension of the vaginal walls, usually accompanied by cystocele/rectocele, makes the lower vagina fuller and therefore better able to provide friction for the penis. What does negatively affect sexuality for the male is vaginal surgery, for it is the elasticity of the vaginal walls that heightens male pleasure. "The elasticity of the vagina is, therefore, important in preserving coital harmony and unnecessary surgical procedures that tend to result in fibrosis and rigidity should be avoided."[10]

Pain with intercourse is not a common complaint amongst prolapsed women. The cause of any true pain should be thoroughly investigated by a qualified physician or women's health care specialist. The cervix, which is easily pushed all the way to the top of the vagina, has many receptors for pressure but should never be painful. In an unhysterectomized woman, a cystocele or rectocele will usually be mild, painless, and responsive to diet, exercise, and discontinuing all straining on the toilet. Adjust to any discomfort by changing position; for example; side-to-side may be more comfortable for women with significant cystocele. Dissection scars however, especially episiotomy and posterior colporraphy scars, will be permanently subject to pain with intercourse. A nourishing herbal salve made of olive oil and beeswax will help keep external tissues pliable and pain free. It is very important that women insist their men understand the history of their injuries and agree on the appropriate amount and frequency of sexual activity. Sex should feel good.

Unless there is some underlying pathology, the nerve stimulation and muscle contraction of sexual activity can only be beneficial in strengthening our natural design. Our emotional reactions to one or more prolapsed organs "getting in the way" of lovemaking are perhaps the greatest barrier to a full and satisfying sexual experience. Actually, it is quite possible that even severe prolapses will remain completely unnoticed by male partners before, during, and after sex. Prolapse is a gravitational problem largely alleviated by lying down. The uterus is repositioned during intercourse and is likely to stay there until we stand up. Even while making love standing or when we are on top, the excitement and movement of sex is likely to keep our pelvic area contracted and "in place." It helps to realize that a cervix prolapsed to the introitus is only a few centimeters lower than normal. With special care, it can be safely managed in this position for a lifetime, or even raised naturally to a more anatomically correct level. The uterus I was once terrified of, I've grown to appreciate as a very tough organ. If given a constant supply of quality nutrition and kept away from deadly pathogens and synthetic chemicals, the uterus is an ally of unsurpassed quality and the keystone to total pelvic health.

✑

Belly Rolls

Belly rolls, an integral part of Middle Eastern dance, are exquisite pelvic floor exercises to perform while having intercourse. Men love them, they feel extraordinarily good to do, and are invaluable for strengthening the entire pelvic area. Think of making a wave beginning at your pubic bone, traveling up to your diaphragm, and back down to your pubis. Do this by pushing your lower belly out, then push your abdomen out. Contract your lower belly, now your abdomen. Do the sequence faster and faster until it forms a continuous wave. Reverse the direction of the wave—abdomen out, lower belly out, abdomen in, lower belly in.

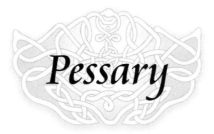

Pessary

Gynecology has become so predominantly a surgical specialty, that one rather hesitates to undertake even a very much qualified defense of such a non-surgical implement as the pessary... The young gynecologist of today frequently has no conception of what the pessary is meant to do and he is apt to be even irritated at the suggestion that such an implement should be accorded at least a modest position in his armamentarium.

EMIL NOVAK, 1923[1]

FITTING THE VAGINA WITH VARIOUS DEVICES to push prolapsed organs back into place is a very old practice. Ancient pessaries were fashioned from linen, wool, hammered brass, waxed cork, and sponges bound with string.[2] Sitz baths using astringent solutions such as pine water and wine to shrink the uterus have also been utilized for millennia.[3,4] Although many women simply live with pelvic organ prolapse, the importance of treating the condition has been known throughout history.

Medical stories hundreds of years old describe cases of complete uterine prolapse (procidentia) that became gangrenous as the uterus strangled outside the vagina.[5] Severe uterine prolapse is also associated with kidney disease caused by constant downward pressure on the ureters, which are embedded in the uterosacral ligaments and transport urine from the kidneys to the bladder.[6] Pelvic organ prolapse is almost always a chronic, non-fatal condition, but as with other degenerative diseases, requires serious effort to stabilize symptoms.

When prolapse becomes symptomatic, a pessary is sometimes prescribed in an attempt to replace the organs in their proper positions. We can be thankful that technology in this area has come a long way since the days of Cleopatra. Today's pessaries are made of the highest-grade silicone. This is not the silicone gel used in breast implants, but a firm, stable, non-reactive, highly biocompatible material. Available in dozens of physician-designed shapes, pessaries can be very effective in relieving symptoms in some women.

High quality silicone pessaries are specially manufactured and can be obtained only by prescription. This alliance between the manufacturer, the distributor (the medical system), and the FDA means you cannot order pessaries directly but must have them ordered for you by your medical doctor.

No studies exist that try to differentiate between those symptoms that can be alleviated by the use of a pessary and those that cannot. There is a lot of anecdotal evidence, however, suggesting that prolapse of the anterior wall is most conducive to pessary use. Some women have reported new-onset rectocele they believe to be associated with pessaries.

Although modern urogynecologists tend to be enthusiastic about fitting their clients with pessaries, for over a century medical doctors have voiced criticism of the pessary based on their own clinical experience. Nichols and Randall stated in 1989 that women

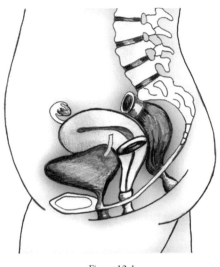

Figure 12-1
Pessary

> Should be advised that the pessary is only palliative, not curative, and acts by continuing a stretch in the opposite direction of tissues that have already been pathologically elongated. Silent progression of the prolapse and widening of the levator hiatus usually will continue until a pessary can no longer be retained.[7]

The observation that pessaries can actually worsen prolapse was made one hundred years earlier, before surgery was a widely accepted option:

> The different kinds of pessaries offered to correct uterine displacement are almost endless. The mere fact that there are so many varieties shows that none yield results quite satisfactorily in actual practice. This conclusion is verified both by the experience of medical men and of suffering patients. We have little to say in their favor and much to say against them. The chief object to be accomplished in curing prolapsus is to restore tone to the vagina by causing it to contract, but if we introduce a pessary of any kind into the passage the genital canal is stretched and its supportive power diminished.[8]

Whether a donut, ring, dish, or Shaatz pessary, the manufacturer's illustrations of how they are supposed to be positioned are all the same and we all try to follow these in-

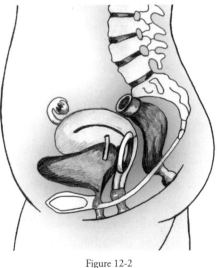

Figure 12-2
Rotated Pessary

structions. The fact that pessaries in this position are holding the upper vagina open and also pressing on the rectum is obvious. (Figure 12-1) However, many women observe that the pessary will flip vertically in order to conform to the natural axis of the vagina (Figure 12-2).

In women with primary prolapse of the anterior wall, a pessary lying more vertically will lift the bladder slightly and improve comfort considerably. A thin pessary such as the ring-with-support will allow the vagina to flatten almost completely. However, for those women with primary prolapse of the central "compartment" the cervix comes down against the rim of the pessary, and if it doesn't push it right out, can be very uncomfortable to wear. Primary prolapse of the posterior wall often negates pessary use entirely.

Stretching of tissues may not be the dynamic responsible for progression of symptoms, but rather that the vagina is held open under intra-abdominal pressure for the other organs to ooze into and fill the void. The vagina's ability to flatten against intra-abdominal pressure made possible full bipedal posture.

જી

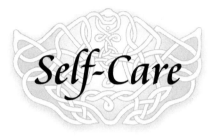

Self-Care

"It is the necessity of my nature to shed all influences."

RALPH WALDO EMERSON[1]

THE INITIAL YEARS AFTER I WAS INFLICTED with uterine prolapse were difficult. I often cried and wished my uterus would go away, until one day when I removed my pessary after having worn it for several hours. A lot of secretions from my uterus had gathered on the pessary and I was curious what they smelled like. To my complete amazement, it was not the briny smell of the vagina, but the exact same smell as baby's breath and fresh, ripe apricots. In an instant I understood the awesome value of my uterus, the necessity of taking special care of it, and the importance of not wishing it away.

I became intently interested in discovering more of its qualities. While I cradled it within me like a precious orb, I began in earnest to exercise and to comprehend which postures lifted and balanced my pelvic system. I paid close attention to which foods seemed to have a salutary effect upon my womb and which aggravated it, causing cramping and heavy menstrual flow.

I became extremely sensitive to pressure or constriction anywhere on my torso. Having grown up in Levi's and T-shirts, it was a bittersweet day when I turned all my old jeans into potholders and placemats. I designed my new wardrobe and breathed a sigh of relief that my pelvic organs were no longer being pushed further "south."

When my uterus felt particularly heavy and uncomfortable, I took sitz baths, placing my perineum into a small tub of warm water to which I added a generous amount of Epsom salts. These mineral salts are composed of magnesium sulfate crystals, which soothe and nourish as they draw out toxins from tissues and organs.

These measures, as well as healing my heart, purifying my environment, and increasing the amount and quality of sleep, all contributed to my beginning to live well with pelvic organ prolapse and to reverse my disease.

In all cases of uterine prolapse, the natural dynamics within the pelvis have shifted so that the uterus is being pushed down into the vagina, like a piston pushing straight down a shaft. The only way to counteract this strong vertical force is to provide as expan-

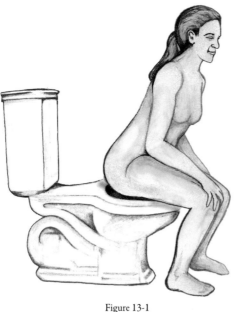

Figure 13-1
Lifting Off the Toilet Seat Into a Half Squat

sive a horizontal plane as possible to diffuse the downward energies. This is accomplished by the Whole Woman Posture™, where a normal lumbar curve is encouraged, while also carrying a solid, round belly in front. In normal anatomy, we carry our bladder, uterus and most of our intestines toward the front of our body. For all women, but particularly women who have given birth, it is simply unnatural to try to attain a flat lower belly and flattened buttocks. Practice the posture as much as possible, while balancing with quality rest and a healthful diet. This really works and you will see that the piston effect of your organs can only go so far because now the downward vertical forces are diffused over a broad horizontal plane. There is now a more supportive internal configuration for the prolapsed uterus, bladder and rectum. Begin to cultivate this "new" image of a healthy, mature female figure, which is actually as old as our original design.

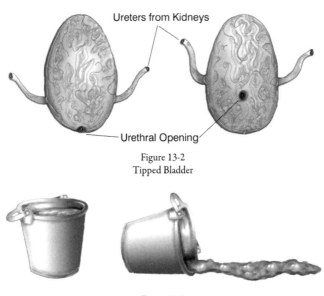

Ureters from Kidneys

Urethral Opening

Figure 13-2
Tipped Bladder

Figure 13-3
Emptying Bladder

If I were healing a cystocele with or without urinary incontinence, my program would be much the same. In addition, I would make sure I completely emptied my bladder every time I urinated. To do this, lift yourself slightly off the toilet seat by rocking forward onto your feet into a half squat (Figure 13-1). This is a more desirable posture for urinating because it places the bladder forward in a more anatomically correct position. Your thigh

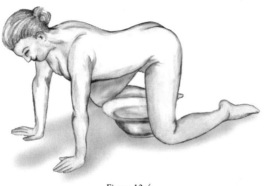

Figure 13-4
Position for Emptying Bladder

muscles will become very strong from supporting you in this natural way. Normally, all urine is emptied from the bladder every time we urinate. The urethra, or outlet of the bladder through which urine exits the body, is found at the bottom or lowest part of the bladder (see left side of Figure 13-2).

With cystocele, however, the bladder has tipped so the opening into the urethra is left higher than the bottom of the bladder (See right side of Figure 13-2). Some urine is now left in the bladder all the time to ferment and cause recurring episodes of cystitis. When we empty a pail of water we turn the pail completely over so the outlet is lower than the bottom of the pail (Figure 13-3). The same is true for the prolapsed bladder. It must be "turned over" at least once a day to allow all urine to empty out.[2] If you continue to have trouble emptying your bladder completely of urine, try urinating on all fours into a shallow basin (Figure 13-4).

If I were healing a rectocele, in addition to a highly energetic diet and quality movement, I would avoid all straining against the toilet seat as in Figure 13-1 and try to sit as much as possible using the strength of my own spine.

I hope it is clear by now that hysterectomy is not a viable solution to any form of prolapse. I am reminded of the childhood game pick-up sticks. As the sticks are thrown, laws of physics and gravity work upon them to a point of stable arrangement. If one stick is removed, chances are dramatically increased that other sticks will fall down.

The pelvic organs are packed tightly together and behave as a single block or unit within the pelvic cavity. Yet, because of natural, fascia-lined spaces between the organs, each can also move and function independently. The uterus forms the hub of a wheel of connective tissue that supports the interior of the pelvis (Figure 13-5). Physiologist and gynecologist Sarah Hackett Stevenson wrote in 1882 of the essential role these structures play in pelvic organ support:

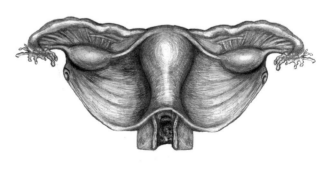

Figure 13-5
Unified Structure of Uterus, Ovaries and Broad Ligaments

> *The most important are called the broad ligaments. They stretch from*
> *each side of the uterus and are attached to the sides of the pelvis in such*
> *a way as to divide the pelvis into two nearly equal parts—the bladder*
> *occupying the front and the rectum the back part of this division.[3]*

When the uterus is removed, a vacuum is created into which fall the bladder, rectum, and bowels. So, too, operations that move pelvic organs into unnatural positions are not viable, nor ones that diminish the nerve supply to pelvic musculature.

Some women prefer the surgical ideal of a "cleaned out" pelvic cavity, whereby problems of prolapse and incontinence are solved for them. They may prefer not to concern themselves much with diet, movement, or a fully active sex life. Women certainly should have this option, but every woman should be made fully aware that once surgery begins, there is no guarantee their pelvic organs, and now their intestinal organs, won't continue an endless descent, requiring repeated surgeries throughout their lifetime.

The natural design of the female spine and pelvis are perfectly adapted to keeping the pelvic organs well positioned over the course of the full human lifespan. Early medical doctors recognized the compromise women have made with civilization:

> *Civilization has done much to elevate woman in the social scale; it has*
> *conferred on her a position quite equal to that enjoyed by man. Civilization*
> *has made woman refined, educated and intellectual; she has been relieved...*
> *from the toilsome drudgery that is regarded by barbarous nations as being*
> *her proper employment. But civilization has not been to woman an unmixed*
> *blessing; it has brought to her very serious drawbacks. Just in proportion as*
> *she has enjoyed the ease, comfort, and luxuries of civilized life, in about*
> *the same ratio she has become afflicted with diseases peculiar to her sex.[4]*

Human females in Western civilization are experiencing a dangerous evolutionary gap. That which at one time was unconscious and instinctive now takes conscious control to maintain. In reality no one can do this work for us. We can travel from physical therapist to chiropractor to urogynecologist and back again, but in the final analysis only we, ourselves can learn to live well moment-to-moment within the natural shape of our original design.

❧

The *Whole Woman* Workout

A TRULY EFFECTIVE TREATMENT PROGRAM must emphasize those same conditions that created our functional design to begin with. At the Whole Woman™ Center we believe prolapse stabilization and reversal to be possible only through a comprehensive restructuring of the entire musculoskeletal system from the ground up. This means no "part" is more important than another and that the whole bodily framework is greater than the sum of its parts in terms of providing pelvic organ support. Central to this restructuring process is the Whole Woman™ Posture. Built upon a scientific framework of natural female growth and development, the Whole Woman™ Posture aims at recreating the structural foundation upon which organ support depends.

Most women in the developed world are fundamentally misshapen, which comes as no surprise given the cultural trappings of our time: baby strollers, play pens, school desks, car seats, couches, chairs, toilets, high heels, and tight clothing. The wide, triangular, primordial human foot has been replaced by narrow feet, pronated ankles, and knocked knees. Long hours in modern work environments have weakened the female shoulder girdle to a point where many women cannot straighten their arms above their head. Likewise, many cannot turn their head to look over their shoulder without significant discomfort. The primal female form has been replaced in our culture by rampant obesity on one hand and anorexic waifs slumping and slouching from movie screens and pages of fashion magazines on the other. Women barely out of their teens show beginning signs of hunchback, while pelvic organ prolapse has become the silent epidemic of our time.

At Whole Woman™ we believe all women can benefit from postural training, and if a woman has all her pelvic organs and is willing to make the effort, almost all cases of prolapse can be positively affected through this work. To call it work is a misnomer however, because it is really joyful human experience to move and live within the natural shape of our original design.

The Whole Woman™ Posture is not something we do once or twice a day, but every time we are on our feet and in sitting positions too. Be sure to balance and support the posture with lots of rest and a high quality diet. This doesn't mean you can never slump into your favorite chair again, but as time goes by that old chair may become less and less inviting. As we assume our natural shape, our old ways of stooping in line at the grocery store or curling up on the sofa just don't feel quite so comfortable anymore.

Meanwhile, prolapse symptoms begin to improve because the muscle and fascial structures attached to our realigned skeleton shift the organs back toward their natural positions. Except in the mildest cases however, this is an incomplete process due to the tendency of pelvic connective tissue to maintain its altered shape, much like a stretched-out sweater. Therefore, many women will experience their conditions stabilizing while also gaining greater strength and flexibility overall.

The natural shape of the female musculoskeleton is re-learned by first assuming the Whole Woman™ Posture. The feet point straight ahead, and it is critical that women understand the importance of keeping this foot alignment with all walking and running activity.

Increasing levels of intensity are utilized to further incorporate the posture into the musculoskeletal framework, and for this we borrow several elements from classical dance. Unlike walking posture, where the feet point straight ahead, the Whole Woman™ Workout is performed with the legs and feet turned out. This is because the ability to externally rotate the femur in the hip joint creates a wider base of support and much greater range of motion from which to bring gravity to bear upon the reshaping process. One set of leg muscles is developed in walking and a different set during the Workout. In this way we provide the best possible structural foundation from which to rebuild our frame.

The Whole Woman™ Workout is joyful, challenging, beneficial movement, yet a wide range of musculoskeletal injuries are possible to sustain if you are not performing this program correctly. That is why it is essential you work slowly, methodically, and intelligently to rebuild your muscles and bones from the arches of your feet to the top of your head. The movements may feel tiring and difficult, but they should never cause pain. If you begin to feel painful sensation—STOP—reevaluate the movement, and begin again only if you are able to identify and correct the source of the discomfort.

The beginning movements look deceptively simple and if they seem easy or boring it means you are not performing them correctly. Please do not continue until you review the instructions given with each movement and feel you fully understand all elements of the exercise.

The workout begins at the ballet barre where we first assess our posture. If you do not have a barre at home, a chair back will substitute. Just be sure the height of the chair back is about at waist level. A series of movements take place at the barre reinforcing every aspect of the postural work by building and stretching the whole body in a highly specific way.

The entire workout is performed barefoot and the importance of stretching and re-building the arches of the feet cannot be overemphasized, as their natural rebound effect relieves from our core abdominal muscles some of the burden of lifting our lower extremities. It is very possible your feet will widen and lengthen with this work, to which the appropriate response would be to fit them with bigger shoes.

From the barre we move into the center of the room where the barre movements are expanded and reinforced through balance and locomotion. Here we use a small wooden baton to stretch and stabilize the arms and shoulders, and correct any "hump" that may have formed in the upper spine.

After 15 minutes of specialized workout the baton is set aside. The session ends with a total body stretch.

The exercises are precisely set to music so that each movement is perfectly matched to musical accompaniment. Listen to the sound of the intro measures, or bars of music, that precede each piece to determine the rhythm of the exercise. Beginning arm and foot positions are given with each lesson. Most of the exercises are performed to the front, side, back, and side.

The Barre

Lesson 1 – The Whole Woman™ Posture

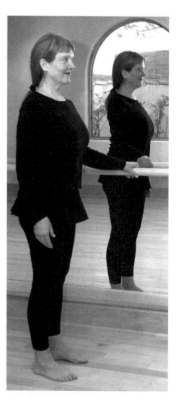

- Begin by placing your left hand on the barre.

- Stand with your feet parallel and approximately six inches apart. Distribute your weight evenly between three points on the soles of your feet: below the big toe, below the little toe, and in the center of the heel.

- Do not roll your ankles in or out. Try to hold them directly over your feet.

- Straighten your knees but do not allow them to bow back. You may have knees that bend to the inside or outside, but the goal is to retrain them so your kneecaps are pointing straight ahead and positioned directly over your ankles.

- Relax your lower belly. Have a sense of pulling up your abdomen from your last pair of ribs. Gently lift your breasts up instead of pulling your belly in.

- Keep your shoulders pressed down. Do not pull them back squeezing your shoulder blades together, but keep your upper back flat and broad.

Figure 14-1
Posture at the Barre

- Pull your head up and forward by slightly tucking your chin. Imagine your whole body being drawn up by a string at the crown of your head.

- This is the posture we are going to maintain during the Whole Woman™ Workout. Throughout each and every movement, a major portion of the exercise is to keep your body in this alignment. It takes a lot of effort and concentration at first, but in time will become very natural.

- As much as possible, breathe in and out through your nose while expanding your lower belly with each inhalation.

Lesson 2 – Positions of the Feet

- First Position. The heels remain together while the toes are turned out approximately 90°. It is critical you understand that turnout does not come from the feet and knees, but is a result of external rotation at the hip joint. If you do not rotate at the hip, great strain is placed on your knees and ankles. If you do rotate at the hip joint, the thigh, knee, ankle, and foot are all in the same alignment as when the feet are parallel. Turnout takes time to develop and we are not striving for the turnout of a ballet dancer, but rather an opening of the lower belly and releasing of the lumbar spine, which happens naturally through this work. Your collarbones and hip crests form two parallel, horizontal lines that should be maintained as much as possible throughout the workout. For instance, when one leg is lifted to the back or side, keeping these two lines parallel will help you not cave in on one side or the other.

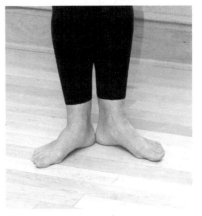

Figure 14-2
Feet in 1st Position

- Second Position. Keeping the same turnout, separate the feet approximately shoulder-width apart. The kneecap should be directly in line with the second and third toes. Make sure your weight is distributed evenly between each foot and that you keep a light touch on the barre.

Lesson 3 – Positions of the Arms

- First Position. The shoulders are held broadly, while the arms form gentle arcs at the sides

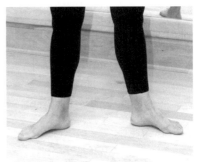

Figure 14-3
Feet in 2nd Position

of the body and the fingertips are placed lightly on the front of each thigh.

- Second Position. The shoulders remain broad, while the arms hold a gentle curve away from and slightly in front of the body. You should be able to see your lower arms and hands from your peripheral vision.

- Fifth Position. The shoulders remain down while the arms and hands are held in an oval above the head. The arms are held slightly forward of the head so your hands are within your peripheral vision.

- Correct use of these arm positions will strengthen the shoulder girdle and reinforce the upper body posture.

- The arm and leg closest to the barre is the *supporting* side, while the arm and leg closest to the center of the room in the *working* side.

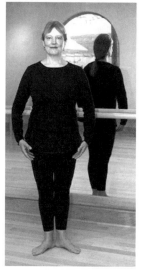
Figure 14-4
Arms 1st Position

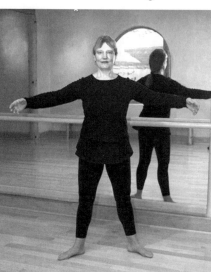
Figure 14-5
Arms 2nd Position

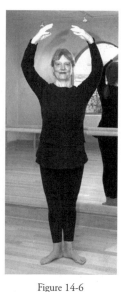
Figure 14-6
Arms 5th Position

Lesson 4 – Head, Shoulder, & Arm Release

Arm Position: 1st
Foot Position: 1st
Music: CD Tracks 1 & 2 – ¾ Slow 64 bars – 2 bar intro

- Place your right hand on the barre.

- Begin to slowly roll your head counterclockwise.

- Take 8 bars of music for one full head circle – to the left, back, right, and front.

- Repeat for another 8 bars.

- Reverse the direction for 2 head circles clockwise using 16 bars of music.

- Make 2 large shoulder rolls using 4 bars of music for each.

- Reverse the shoulder rolls for another 8 bars.

- Using 4 bars of music, while keeping your shoulders down, gracefully raise your arm up and out to the side leading with your elbow and followed by wrist and fingertips to end with your arm stretched overhead.

- Lower your arm for 4 bars leading with your elbow and followed by your wrist and then fingertips.

- Repeat the arm raise for another 8 bars.

- Turn around and place your left hand on the barre to repeat this entire sequence.

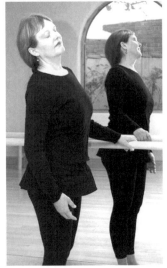
Figure 14-7
Head Roll

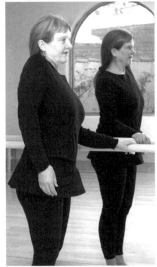
Figure 14-8
Shoulder Roll

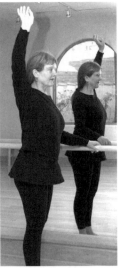
Figure 14-9
Arm Raise

Lesson 5 – Plié

Arm Position: 1st
Foot Position: 1st
Music: CD Tracks 3 & 4 – 4/4 Slow 32 bars – 2 bar intro

- Place your right hand on the barre.

- Beginning in 1st position and keeping knees over the second and third toes, bend straight down as far as you can go while keeping your heels on the floor. This movement warms up the thighs and buttocks, while stretching the muscles of the calf.

- Perform 4 pliés in 1st position using 4 bars of music each.

- Without skipping a beat, open arms and feet out to 2nd position and bend the knees, always keeping them directly over the toes. Consciously tighten your pelvic diaphragm as you rise out of plié and sense your pelvic organs shifting up and forward over your pubic bone.

- Perform 4 pliés in 2nd position for a total of 16 bars of music.

- The plié forms the basis of the Whole Woman™ Workout; it is very important that you understand and perform it well. At first it is a part of our warm up, but later will become the cushion necessary for more rigorous movement.

- Turn around and place your left hand on the barre to repeat this entire sequence.

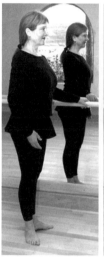
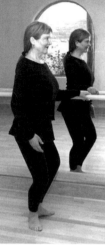
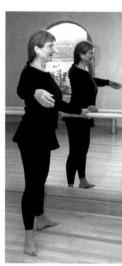
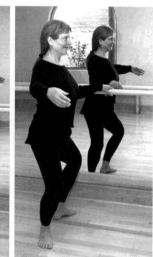

| Figure 14-10 | Figure 14-11 | Figure 14-12 | Figure 14-13 |
| Plié 1st Position Start | Plié 1st Position | Plié 2nd Position Start | Plié 2nd Position |

Lesson 6 – Tendu

Arm Position: 2nd
Foot Position: 1st
Music: CD Tracks 5 & 6 – 6/8 Moderate 32 bars – 2 bar intro

- Place your right hand on the barre.

- Tendu rhymes with fondue and means "to stretch." This is a stretch of the working foot to the front, side, back, and side.

- Beginning in 1st position, the working foot brushes along the floor toward the front as it extends through the arch, metatarsals, and toes to a full point.

- Create resistance by slightly pushing into the floor as the foot brushes forward. Stretch the toes as much as possible during the full point, and again create resistance in the metatarsals as the foot returns to 1st position.

- Brush out to the side in the same manner; to the back, and again to the side.

- Take 2 bars of music to stretch the foot out and 2 bars to return, for a total of 4 sets of tendu to the front, side, back, and side.

- Tendu increases strength and flexibility in the foot arches.

- Tendu is also a very good exercise to reinforce hip turnout. If you are properly turned out at the hip joint as your foot stretches toward the back, the top of your working foot should be facing out toward the center of the room and not toward the floor.

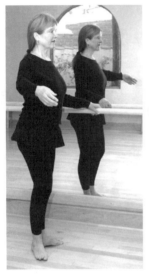

Figure 14-14
Tendu Start

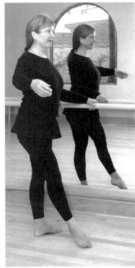

Figure 14-15
Tendu Front

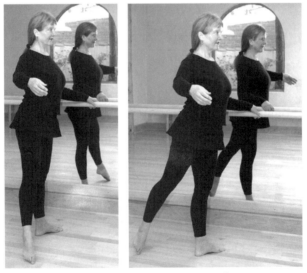

Figure 14-16
Tendu Side

Figure 14-17
Tendu Back

- Remember to pull up out of the supporting hip. The goal is to have all aspects of your posture stay the same, except the working leg.

- Turn around and place your left hand on the barre to repeat this sequence.

Lesson 7 – Point & Flex; Ankle Circles

Arm Position: 2nd
Foot Position: 1st
Music: CD Tracks 7 & 8 – 6/8 Moderate 32 bars – 2 bar intro

- Place your right hand on the barre.

- Beginning in 1st position brush to the front, raising your foot slightly off the floor and coming to a full point. Follow by flexing the foot to its fullest. Perform 16 sets of point/flex for a total of 16 bars.

- Without skipping a beat, begin to circle clockwise at the ankle joint and continue for another 8 bars of music. Reverse the circles for the last 8 bars.

- This exercise strengthens and makes more flexible the structures of the foot and ankle.

- Turn around and place your left hand on the barre to repeat this sequence.

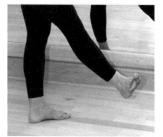
Figure 14-18
Point

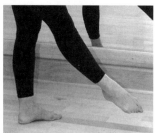
Figure 14-19
Flex

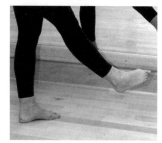
Figure 14-20
Circle

Lesson 8 – Tendu With Plié

Arm Position: 2nd
Foot Position: 1st
Music: CD Tracks 9 & 10 – 2/4 Moderate 64 bars – 4 bar intro

- Place your right hand on the barre.

- Beginning in 1st position, tendu to the front to a full point. Returning to 1st, come immediately down into plié while keeping your heels on the floor.

- As you rise from plié, tendu out to the side. Return to plié and do the same to the back and again to the side. Keep the motion fluid as you pull up into the posture. Shoulders down; chin slightly tucked.

- Each tendu/plié takes 4 bars of music for a total of 4 sets.

- Turn around and place your left hand on the barre to repeat this sequence.

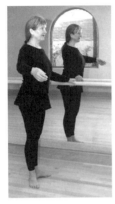

Figure 14-21
Tendu with Plié Start

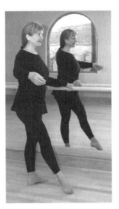

Figure 14-22
Tendu Front

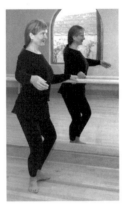

Figure 14-23
Plié

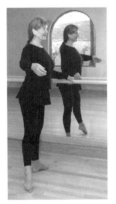

Figure 14-24
Tendu Side

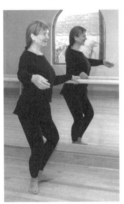

Figure 14-25
Plié

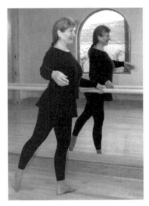

Figure 14-26
Tendu Back

Lesson 9 – Leg Lifts

Arm Position: 2nd
Foot Position: 1st
Music: CD Tracks 11 & 12 – 3/4 Moderate 64 bars – 4 bar intro

- Place your right hand on the barre.

- Beginning in 1st position, lift your leg to the front until you feel both resistance and a gentle stretch in your hamstring muscles. Close back to 1st.

- This is a slow, controlled leg lift and there should be no flopping of the leg or foot during the lift or with closure. Remember not to collapse on the supporting side, but to keep pulling up through the posture. Only the lower extremity moves. The torso must stay completely stationary.

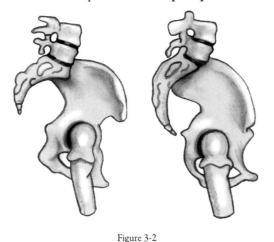